Normal and Disordered Phonology in Children

Child Language Acquisition Series

Published Titles

Mabel L. Rice, Ph.D., and Susan Kemper, Ph.D. *Child Language and Cognition: Contemporary Issues* (1984)

Titles in Preparation

Marion Blank, Ph.D., et al. *Developmental Discourse Therapy: Using Basic Research for Effective Intervention*

Stan A. Kuczaj II, Ph.D. *Children's Acquisition of Word Meanings*

Helen Tager-Flusberg, Ph.D. *The Acquisition of Syntax*

Ina Č. Užgiris, Ph.D. *Communication: The Foundation for Language*

 A University Park Press
Topicbook

The University Park Press Topicbooks are carefully selected, written, and designed to identify the issues and controversies in communication science and disorders, to help readers find their way through the broad range of information available, and to serve as short topical introductions for professionals and students.

A volume in the Child Language Acquisition Series

Normal and Disordered Phonology in Children

Carol Stoel-Gammon, Ph.D.
Department of Speech and Hearing Sciences
University of Washington

Carla Dunn, Ph.D.
Department of Speech Communication
University of Texas at Austin

University Park Press • Baltimore

University Park Press
International Publishers in Medicine and Allied Health
300 North Charles Street
Baltimore, Maryland 21201

Sponsoring editor: Janet S. Hankin
Production editor: Megan Barnard Shelton
Cover and text design by: Caliber Design Planning, Inc.
Series logo by: Barry Goldman Designs

Typeset by: Waldman Graphics, Inc.
Manufactured in the United States of America by: Halliday Lithograph

Library of Congress Cataloging in Publication Data

Stoel-Gammon, Carol.
  Normal and disordered phonology in children.

  "A volume in the child language acquisition series."
  Includes index.
  1. Speech disorders in children. 2. English language—
Phonology. I. Dunn, Carla. II. Title. [DNLM: 1. Phonetics. 2. Speech—physiology. 3. Speech Disorders—in
infancy & childhood. 4. Speech—in infancy & childhood.
WS   105.5.C8   S872N]
RJ496.S7S79   1984   618.92′85′5   84-15309
ISBN 0-8391-1871-6

To Richard, Daniel, and Kate Gammon

To Margaret and Carlos Dunn

Contents

Preface to the *Child Language Acquisition* Series

The study of child language acquisition has emerged, in the past 15 years, as a distinct and rapidly growing field of inquiry, located at the intersection of several established disciplines. The books included in the *Child Language Acquisition* series cover key topics in this growing and diverse literature. The goal of each volume is to summarize the research knowledge of a particular aspect of language acquisition, synthesizing different theoretical perspectives and academic disciplines. Within each volume the range of children's achievement of language acquisition is addressed, from the apparently effortless mastery by normally developing children to the limited or unusual language acquired by atypical children.

The books are written for advanced undergraduate and graduate students as well as for professionals providing service to children and researchers in related disciplines. Each volume is written at an introductory level, with clear definitions of terms, substantive discussions of major theoretical and empirical issues, and judicious referencing of original sources. The topics will include the sources of language (biological, cognitive, social, and environmental), aspects of language (phonology, word meaning, grammar, and discourse), and patterns of atypical acquisition (developmental language disorders, learning disabilities, mental retardation, deafness, and bilingualism). The books can be grouped or used individually in courses covering such topics as child language acquisition, cognitive development, social development, and education of young children.

Normal and Disordered Phonology in Children, by Stoel-Gammon and Dunn, provides an unusually comprehensive and balanced account of children's phonological development. It reflects major theoretical innovations in the study of phonology, such as process analysis, while clearly presenting the utility of traditional concepts such as phonemes and distinctive features. Phonological development is set into a broader framework including other aspects of language, as well as underlying perceptual and cognitive processes. The authors' approach is sensitive to the substantial individual differences among normally developing and language-disordered children, and the resulting need to tailor assessment as well as intervention procedures to individual children. Particular attention is paid to the advantages and problems of the various methodologies of studying and assessing phonological development. This clear and comprehensive "state of the art" in phonological development provides a sound basis for clinical and educational practice, as well as providing a framework for continuing research in this area.

Preface

The field of child phonology has expanded rapidly during the past decade. Not only has the amount of research increased dramatically, the scope of study has become much broader, encompassing the work of investigators from a variety of disciplines and permitting collaboration between investigators from different backgrounds. This book is the result of one such collaboration; the two authors, both interested in child phonology (but from somewhat different points of view), come from two disciplines: one was trained as a linguist, the other as a speech-language pathologist.

The goal of the book is to integrate the knowledge from both disciplines, specifically to: (1) review and critique the current body of literature on normal and disordered phonological development in children and (2) relate the current research in child phonology to the clinical issues of assessment and treatment of children with phonological disorders. The book is intended for students of linguistics, speech-language pathology, early childhood education, and child development. It is assumed that the readers have a basic understanding of phonetics and phonology.

As we finish the project, there are several people whose help and encouragement we would like to acknowledge.

First, we want to thank each other for the thoughtfulness, enthusiasm, and dedication given to the project. Neither of us had anticipated the amount of time and energy this book would require.

Second, we want to acknowledge the help of our friends and colleagues who listened to, read, discussed, and critiqued our ideas during the preparation of the manuscript. In particular, Mary Coberly, Barbara Bain, and Laurie Newton deserve to be mentioned in this regard.

Third, we never could have finished without the help of Jane Creazzi, Katie King, and Debbie Bryant, the skilled and patient typists who were there when we needed them.

A special acknowledgment is due to Philip Dale, who read and critiqued various drafts of the manuscript. His insightful comments were particularly valuable in allowing us to place our material in the broader framework of child development.

Finally, we want to thank all the children whose speech appears in the chapters that follow. Without them, we would have had little to say.

Carol Stoel-Gammon

Carla Dunn

Chapter 1

Introduction

Babies begin to coo and babble shortly after birth. They produce identifiable words around their first birthday and short sentences around their second birthday. By the age of five, they have acquired a vocabulary of about 2,000 words, can produce syntactically complex sentences, and can accurately pronounce a majority of the sounds of their language; they are, in essence, well on their way to full mastery of the structural and pragmatic aspects of one of the most complex communication systems we know—human language. These are the facts. The related question is: How do children go about learning to talk? How do they learn to combine sound and meaning to form words? To join words together to make sentences? To use sentences appropriately to make statements, ask questions, and converse with those around them? Although most children have acquired much of the adult linguistic system by the age of five, some have not. For these children, we must ask: Why did they fail to learn language as their peers did? What can be done about it?

These are questions that have fascinated people from all walks of life for centuries, and during the past few decades the fascination has increased as we have come to understand more and more about human language behavior in general and language acquisition in particular. The recent advances in our knowledge can be attributed to a number of factors ranging from the introduction of new linguistic theories, to technological advances in the instrumentation used for the collection and analysis of language samples, to contributions of researchers and scholars from a variety of disciplines including linguistics, philosophy, psychology, education, speech science, and communication disorders.

This book focuses on an area that has benefited immensely from the broadened perspective of language learning: child phonology. As Jenkins stated in the concluding remarks of a child phonology conference in 1978, this is an area of study that is "fresh, young, and rapidly expanding" with much of the research carried out during the last decade (Jenkins, 1980). Papers read at the 1978 conference (published in 1980; see Yeni-Komshian, Kavanagh, and Ferguson) covered a diverse set of topics, including infant speech perception, infant vocalizations, cross-linguistic studies of phonological theory, the development of phonological rhythm, speech perception of language-delayed children, and the relationship between perception and production, to name a few. The scope of topics discussed reveals the broad-based approach now being taken to the study of child phonology.

Until the 1970s, the field was much narrower in terms of the disciplines involved and the issues of interest. The majority of research was done by linguists (e.g., Leopold, 1947) who were primarily interested in studying the order of acquisition of phonemes and phonemic contrasts in order to determine which phonological theory would best predict and explain the order. Speech-language pathologists and educators (e.g., Templin, 1957) were also interested in studies of phonemic acquisition but for a different reason. They wanted to know the *age* at which the various phonemes were acquired (i.e., produced correctly) so that they could identify those children who were falling behind the age-appropriate norms.

The emphasis on studying the order of acquisition of phonemes can be attributed to the influence of Roman Jakobson, a linguist whose pioneering monograph published in 1941 (English translation, 1968) postulated a relationship between phonological development in children, phonological universals of the languages of the world, and phonological loss resulting from aphasia. According to Jakobson, children's vocal productions can be divided into two periods, babbling and meaningful speech; the periods are characterized as being distinct from each other with little or no relationship between them. During the prelinguistic period, the vocalizations are said to be "ephemeral" and "random" and do not conform to any developmental pattern. In contrast, after the onset of "true speech," phonemic development is said to follow a universal and innate order regulated by a hierarchical set of structural laws (Jakobson, 1968).

Jakobson's monograph and subsequent writings (Jakobson, 1971; Jakobson and Halle, 1956) had two major effects on the field of child phonology. First, they established child phonology as a legitimate area of linguistic study and inspired a series of studies aimed at determining if the postulated order of phonemic acquisition was in fact supported by data from studies of children acquiring different languages (e.g., Leopold, 1947; Nakazima, 1962; Pačesova, 1968; Velten, 1943). Second, Jakobson's statements regarding babbling and its (non)relationship to meaningful speech tended to discourage linguists and phonologists from studying infant vocal productions during the prelinguistic period because it was assumed they played a minimal role in subsequent phonological development.

Although Jakobson's theory continues to be influential, alternative theories of phonological development were introduced during the 1970s, causing researchers to investigate issues other than the order of acquisition of phonemes. In addition, the role of babbling was reexamined (Locke, 1983b; Oller et al., 1976) and was found to be more closely related to the phonology of early meaningful speech than had previously been thought. At present, the study of child phonology benefits from the input of scholars trained in a variety of disciplines, including linguistics, psychology, speech science, and speech-language pathology. The aim of this book is to provide an overview of our current knowledge of phonological development in children, with particular emphasis on the work carried out during the past 10–15 years. The book focuses on normal phonological development and its relationship to the study of disordered phonology in children. Throughout the text, the importance of viewing normal development as a basis for understanding disorders is emphasized.

Although some researchers speak of "articulatory acquisition" (e.g., Winitz, 1969) and "articulatory disorders" (e.g., Shelton and McReynolds, 1979), we believe that *phonological acquisition* and *phonological disorder* are more appropriate terms. In our view, "articulation" refers to the physical movements involved in the production of speech, whereas "phonology" has two broader meanings. In one sense, it refers to the organization and classification of speech sounds that occur as contrastive units within a given language, and in another sense it is used as a general term referring to *all* aspects of the study of speech sounds, including speech perception and production, as well as cognitive and motor aspects of speech. We, along with other researchers in the field (e.g., Ferguson and Yeni-Komshian, 1980; Grunwell, 1982; Shriberg, 1982a), have adopted this broader definition of phonology in our discussion of phonological development in children.

Given the definition outlined above, it follows that articulatory acquisition is part of phonological development—that part that involves mastery of the motor ability to accurately produce the sounds and sound sequences of the adult language. In acquiring adult-like articulatory patterns, the child must learn to control the flow of air from the lungs through the larynx in order to produce voiced and voiceless sounds, the opening and closing of the velopharyngeal port to produce oral and nasal sounds, and the movement of the tongue, lips, and jaw to produce the various consonant and vowel sounds of the language.

In addition to the physical movements involved in speech production, the organizational (or structural) aspects of the sound system of the language must also be learned. For example, children must figure out: (1) which sound differences are contrastive and which are not; (2) what kinds of positional and sequential constraints are placed on the various speech sounds (e.g., in English, the phoneme /ʒ/ does not occur at the beginning of words, /h/ does not occur at the end); and (3) what rules, or processes, are involved with the morphophonemic alternations of the language (e.g., in English, the final /t/ of *hit* and *eat* is produced as a flap [ɾ] when it precedes an unstressed vowel as in *hitter* [hɪɾɚ] and *eating* [iɾɪŋ]).

The study of child phonology, then, covers a broad range of behaviors and can be approached from a variety of disciplines— audiology, acoustics, child development, psycholinguistics, speech perception, and speech-language pathology, to name a few. In this volume, we briefly address a number of topics but have chosen to concentrate on only a few. In the chapters that follow, we focus more on *production* than on perception, on *segmental* more than suprasegmental aspects, on the *linguistic* rather than the *prelinguistic* stage, on phonological acquisition of *American English* rather than of other languages, and on *perceptual* (i.e., transcription-based) rather than acoustic studies. The discussion of disordered phonology is limited to children who have no identifiable etiology, i.e., children who have traditionally been referred to as having "functional articulation disorders" (Powers, 1957). However, the principles of assessment and remediation presented in Chapters 6 and 7 can be adapted to apply to other populations, e.g., cleft palate, hearing impaired, mentally retarded. It is assumed in these chapters that readers are familiar with traditional techniques of assessment (e.g., Templin and Darley, 1960) and remediation (Van Riper, 1972; Winitz, 1969) of phonological disorders.

Current Issues

During the last decade, investigations of phonological development have gone beyond the question of order of acquisition of phonemes to a broader range of issues. The major issues, as we see them, are briefly described below and are discussed in the chapters that follow. It is not our intention to provide hard-and-fast answers to any of the questions outlined here, but to review the relevant literature and attempt to construct a framework that allows the issues to be considered from various points of view.

Universal Patterns Versus Individual Differences

Simply put, this issue centers around the question: Does phonological development proceed along a universal, and presumably, innate, course or does each child follow his or her own idiosyncratic path? The issue has become a central one in current theories of phonological acquisition, because it separates the universalist theories (e.g., Jakobson, 1968; Stampe, 1969, 1973) from the more cognitively based theories (e.g., Macken and Ferguson, 1983; Waterson, 1971).

Research suggests that there is no simple answer to the question. It seems that some aspects of acquisition are universal or near-universal (e.g., the predominant sounds and syllable types of babbling), whereas others are subject to considerable variation (e.g., the order of acquisition of phonemes and phonemic contrasts). Given the existence of individual differences, it is important to try to delimit the normal range of differences so we can identify those children who fall outside that range, i.e., children who are *not* developing normally.

Factors Underlying Mispronunciations

One does not have to be a linguist or a speech-language pathologist to recognize pronunciation errors in a young child's speech.

Such errors occur commonly in a normally developing 2-year-old (or an older phonologically disordered child) and are easily identified by most adults and older children. The difficult part about mispronunciations is determining *why* they occur. There are several possible causes ranging from physical to perceptual to cognitive; these include: (1) lack of motor ability to *articulate* a sound or sequence of sounds; (2) failure to *perceive* a word accurately; (3) failure to *remember* (i.e., store) the pronunciation accurately; (4) a *production constraint* on the general form of all words (e.g., no word can end in a consonant); (5) a *lack of knowledge* about the phonological system of the adult language (e.g., the child may not "know" that /s/ and /ʃ/ are distinct phonemes in English and consequently might treat them as variants of a single phoneme); and (6) any combination of the above. This list is not intended to be exhaustive but to illustrate the range of factors that must be considered when trying to determine the cause(s) of a pronunciation error. For clinical purposes, it is particularly important to identify the factors underlying production errors in order to determine the most effective treatment plan.

Units of Acquisition

For many years the *unit* of acquisition was never questioned. It was simply assumed that children acquired phonemes and contrasts between phonemes (i.e., distinctive features). There is now a body of research that suggests that this is not the case. In the early stages it seems that children learn whole words (Ferguson and Farwell, 1975) or even phrases (Peters, 1983) rather than phonemes or features (Jakobson, 1968). The transition from whole words to phonemes does not occur abruptly, and thus some words may be learned as indivisible wholes at the same time that others are acquired as sequences of phonemes.

The issue of units of acquisition is particularly important when selecting appropriate techniques for analyzing a given child's speech. If a child is at the stage of learning words as indivisible wholes, it is obvious that analysis in terms of distinctive features will not tell us much about his/her phonological system. Conversely, a lexical (or word-by-word) analysis is not adequate for children in the phonemic stage. Consideration of units is also important for remediation, because the units that are selected to be taught (e.g., features, isolated sounds, syllables, words) influence treatment results.

Nature of Disordered Phonology

A major difficulty in talking about *disordered phonology* in children is defining what constitutes a disorder (Grunwell, 1981). Are the phonological characteristics of children with a disorder essentially the same as those of young normally developing children or are they qualitatively different? In other words, are the children best described as *delayed* because their pronunciations evidence characteristics typically found in the speech of much younger children, or should they be described as *deviant* because their pronunciation patterns do not occur in normally developing children?

A related question concerns the children themselves: Do children assessed as having a phonological disorder form a homogeneous group, or are there identifiable subgroups based, perhaps, on different etiologies? It could be, for example, that some children are "delayed" and others are "deviant" in their phonological development.

Generalization

In discussions of phonological disorders, *generalization* is cited as one of the important goals of remediation. Although the term "generalization" has been used in a variety of ways, in most cases it seems to refer to one of two basic types of learning. In the first type, generalization is said to occur when sounds are produced correctly in new phonetic contexts (e.g., /s/ is produced correctly in final position after being trained in initial position) or in new communicative settings (e.g., /s/ is produced at home after training in the clinic). In the second type, generalization is said to occur when untrained sounds or syllabic shapes are produced correctly after training on phonetically similar sounds or syllables (e.g., /s/ is produced correctly after training on /z/).

Obviously, generalization is a desirable goal for remediation because, if it does not occur, every sound (or distinctive feature) must be taught in every phonetic context and every communicative setting. One problem with assuming that generalization is easily achieved is that studies of young children developing normally suggest that generalization of a sound or a feature to new phonetic contexts is limited. Phonemes are often learned in one position first and considerably later in others; and although some features (e.g., nasality) may be acquired "across-the-board," others (e.g., sibilance) appear first in a few sounds, later in others. Given this information about normal acquisition, we should not simply assume that disordered children generalize their training without special assistance. If generalization is to be a viable goal, two questions must be addressed: (1) How can generalization be achieved most efficiently in treatment? (2) Why does generalization seem to occur rapidly in some disordered children but is limited or nonexistent in others?

Concepts and Terms

Phonetic Features

In the chapters that follow, speech sounds are represented by phonetic symbols and referred to using phonetic terms. It is assumed that the reader has at the least a working knowledge of the articulatory features used to describe the phonemes of English. Tables 1.1 and 1.2 present the symbols and general features we use when discussing the consonantal and vocalic systems of American English. A more comprehensive chart of phonetic symbols and articulatory features appears in Appendix A.

Analysis of Speech Sounds

There are two main types of analysis of speech production, commonly referred to as *phonetic* and *phonological*. A phonetic analysis provides a detailed description of speech sounds, or *phones*, in terms of their articulatory, acoustic, and psychoacoustic, or auditory, properties. *Articulatory phonetics* is concerned with the way in which speech is produced by the vocal mechanism, *acoustic phonetics* with the physical properties of speech sounds, and *psychoacoustics* with the way in which speech sounds are perceived by the listener. In contrast to phonetic analyses, which are purely descriptive, a *phonological analysis* is concerned with the classification and organization of speech sounds that occur as contrastive units, or *phonemes*, in a given language. The goal of a phonological analysis is to determine the inventory of phonemes in a language and to describe their patterns of occurrence. A phonological analysis

Table 1.1 Articulatory Features of the Consonantal Phonemes of English

Feature	Bilabial	Labiodental	Interdental	Alveolar	Palatal	Velar	Glottal
Nasal	m			n		ŋ	
Stop							
Voiceless	p			t		k	ʔ
Voiced	b			d		g	
Fricative							
Voiceless		f	θ	s	ʃ		
Voiced		v	ð	z	ʒ		
Affricate							
Voiceless					tʃ		
Voiced					dʒ		
Glide							
Voiceless							
Voiced	w				j		h
Liquid							
Rhotic				r			
Lateral				l			

Table 1.2 Articulatory Features of the Vowels of American English

Feature	Front	Central	Back
High			
Tense	i		u
Lax	ɪ		ʊ
Mid			
Tense	e		o
Lax	ɛ	ə ʌ	ɔ
Low			
Tense		a	
Lax	æ		

of English, for example, would include statements of the following type:

1. The phoneme /ŋ/ occurs in word-medial and word-final position, but never in word-initial position.
2. The phoneme /h/ occurs in word-initial position and medially between vowels, but never in word-final position.
3. If a word begins with a sequence of three consonants, the first is /s/, the second is /p/, /t/, or /k/, and the third /r/, /l/, /w/, or /j/.

In addition to a phonemic inventory, a phonological analysis must include a description of the phonemes as they are pronounced in various phonetic contexts. In many instances a single phoneme has more than one pronunciation. Consider, for example, the pronunciation of the phoneme /k/ in the words *key* and *coo*. In *key*, /k/ is articulated with tongue contact toward the front of the mouth; in *coo*, tongue contact is further back. Variants of a single phoneme, such as these two pronunciations of /k/, are called *allophones*.

Allophones of a single phoneme may be in *complementary distribution* or in *free variation*. If they are in complementary distribution, they never occur in exactly the same phonetic context. For example, in English, the phoneme /p/ in initial position has two allophones: it is aspirated (produced [pʰ]) when it precedes a vowel, e.g., pie [pʰaɪ]; it is unaspirated when it precedes /l/ or /r/, e.g., pry [praɪ], ply [plaɪ]. Allophones in free variation can occur in the same phonetic context. In English, the phoneme /p/ in final position has allophones that are in free variation; in the word *up*, for example, /p/ may be released with a small burst of air as the lips open, [pʰ], or unreleased if lip closure is maintained, [p˥].

In addition to descriptions of allophonic variation, a phonological analysis includes statements regarding *morphophonemic alternation*. In English there would be a statement defining the relationship between the word-final [k] of *electric* and *public* and the morpheme-final [s] of *electricity* and *publicity*, or between the final [n] of *sign* and *resign* and the sequence [gn] of *signature* and *resignation*. In sum, a phonological analysis includes: (1) a description of the phonemes of the language; (2) statements regarding positional and sequential restrictions on occurrence; and (3) descriptions of allophonic and morphophonemic variation.

Distinctive Features

So far the discussion has focused entirely on phonemes; and although phonemes are basic units in any phonological analysis, phonemic systems are often described in terms of *distinctive features*. In such descriptions, each phoneme is analyzed as a "bundle" of distinctive features and is distinguished from all other phonemes by its unique combination of features. Consider the following fricative phonemes of English:

Labiodental	Interdental	Alveolar	Palatal
/f, v/	/θ, ð/	/s, z/	/ʃ, ʒ/

In each pair, the phonemes are distinguished by a single distinctive feature—voicing; the first member of the pair is voiceless, the second is voiced.

Distinctive features can be used to group phonemes into classes on the basis of shared features. In English, for example, the phonemes /m,n,ŋ/ share the feature *nasal* and thus form a class of nasal consonants; all other consonants are non-nasal (or oral). When a group of phonemes can be described by fewer distinctive features than any of its members, those phonemes are said to form a *natural class*. Thus the phonemes /m,n,ŋ/ make up the natural class of *nasals*.

The concept of natural class has proved useful in phonological analysis because phonemes grouped into natural classes tend to be organized in similar patterns in the phonological system of a language. For example, it was noted above that /p/ in initial position has two allophones: It was aspirated before a vowel but unaspirated before /l/ or /r/. Further examination of the sound pattern of English reveals that the phonemes /t/ and /k/ evidence the same type of allophonic variation—they are aspirated before vowels and unaspirated before /l/ and /r/ (the sequence /tl/ does not occur word initially). In articulatory terms, phonemes /p, t, k/ share features of manner and voicing: they are all voiceless stops and thus form a natural class. All three members of this class display the same types of allophonic variation in word-initial and word-final position described for /p/ in the preceding paragraphs, thereby permitting a single statement to describe the behavior of the entire class. It is evident from this example that description in terms of features and natural classes facilitate analysis of a sound system by permitting phonological patterns to be stated in general terms.

Although there is general agreement that a distinctive feature system should consist of a universal set of features that describe the phonemic systems of all the languages of the world, there is as yet no consensus as to the number and type of features that belong in that universal set. The first system to be widely used was developed during the 1950s by Jakobson et al. (1963; see also Jakobson and Halle, 1956). The system consisted of 12 binary features defined by their acoustic and articulatory properties. Feature systems that have been developed more recently, e.g., those of Chomsky and Halle (1968) and Ladefoged (1971, 1975), have included more distinctive features, nearly 30 (in contrast to 12), and have been based for the most part on articulatory dimensions. Like the system of Jakobson et al. (1963), the Chomsky-Halle feature set consisted of *binary* features, meaning that for any given segment a feature was either present or absent. In contrast, Ladefoged (1971) incorporated both binary and multivalued features into his system, arguing that multivalued features were necessary because nearly all languages use at least two features in a nonbinary way: *articulatory place* (e.g., labial, labiodental, dental, alveolar), which may have as many as six values in a given language, and *vowel height*, which may have as many as four values (high, mid-high, mid-low, low).

Although a number of studies of child speech have used the Chomsky-Halle feature system (Compton, 1970; McReynolds and Huston, 1971), it is our opinion that a feature system based primarily on articulatory properties is more appropriate, particularly if the goal of the analysis is a clinical description of disordered phonology (see Chapter 6). The system we have developed is presented in Table 1.3. Although the consonantal system can be defined by fewer features, we have found that each of the features listed is useful in describing some aspect of a developing or disordered phonological system.

An understanding of the terminology and concepts described above is a necessary prerequisite to the study of normal phonological development and disordered phonology. Readers who be-

Table 1.3 Feature Specifications for the Consonantal Phonemes of English

	p	b	t	d	k	g	ʔ	m	n	ŋ	f	v	θ	ð	s	z	ʃ	ʒ	tʃ	dʒ	l	r	w	j	h
Consonantal	+	+	+	+	+	+	+	+	+	+	+	+	+	+	+	+	+	+	+	+	+	+	−	−	−
Sonorant	−	−	−	−	−	−	−	+	+	+	−	−	−	−	−	−	−	−	−	−	+	+	+	+	−
Voiced	−	+	−	+	−	+	−	+	+	+	−	+	−	+	−	+	−	+	−	+	+	+	+	+	−
Nasal	−	−	−	−	−	−	−	+	+	+	−	−	−	−	−	−	−	−	−	−	−	−	−	−	−
Continuant	−	−	−	−	−	−	−	−	−	−	+	+	+	+	+	+	+	+	−	−	+	+	+	+	+
Strident	−	−	−	−	−	−	−	−	−	−	+	+	−	−	+	+	+	+	+	+	−	−	−	−	−
Lateral	−	−	−	−	−	−	−	−	−	−	−	−	−	−	−	−	−	−	−	−	+	−	−	−	−
Labial	+	+	−	−	−	−	−	+	−	−	+	+	−	−	−	−	−	−	−	−	−	−	+	−	−
Alveolar	−	−	+	+	−	−	−	−	+	−	−	−	+	+	+	+	−	−	−	−	+	+	−	−	−
Palatal	−	−	−	−	−	−	−	−	−	−	−	−	−	−	−	−	+	+	+	+	−	−	−	+	−
Velar	−	−	−	−	+	+	−	−	−	+	−	−	−	−	−	−	−	−	−	−	−	−	+	−	−
Glottal	−	−	−	−	−	−	+	−	−	−	−	−	−	−	−	−	−	−	−	−	−	−	−	−	+

lieve their background in phonetics and phonology is inadequate may want to supplement the review presented in this chapter with other readings in the area. Possible references include the books by Ladefoged (1975) and Tiffany and Carrell (1977) for phonetics, and Hyman (1975) and Sloat et al. (1978) for phonology.

Conclusion

This book provides an overview of phonological development and relates our understanding of normal development to the study of phonological disorders in children. Chapter 2 deals with the course of phonological development from the prelinguistic period through the acquisition of the adult phonemic system with particular attention to the early stages of linguistic development (i.e., 12–48 months). Chapter 3 discusses the process of acquisition, and Chapter 4 is devoted to a discussion of methods currently used in the study of phonological development. The next three chapters focus on aspects of disordered phonology: the nature of disorders (Chapter 5), clinical assessment of children with a disorder (Chapter 6), and principles and techniques of remediation (Chapter 7). The final chapter presents a summary of the major issues discussed and provides suggestions for future topics of study.

Chapter 2

Normal Phonological Development

The discussion of normal phonological development is divided into two parts, dealing with two interdependent aspects of acquisition. The first part (presented in this chapter) focuses on observable phenomena, i.e., the *product* of acquisition, and the second part (Chapter 3) deals with aspects that are not directly observable, i.e., the *process* of acquisition. The purpose of the present chapter is to provide a description of the speech sounds produced, the approximate ages and stages of phonological development, and the common error patterns occurring in meaningful speech. Much has been written on these topics, particularly during the past decade, making it impossible to cover all facets in depth. As mentioned earlier, we have chosen to give more attention to the stage of meaningful speech than to babbling, to production than to perception, and to segmental (primarily consonantal) than to suprasegmental acquisition. An overview of the stages of normal development is presented first to provide a general framework for the more detailed discussions that follow.

Stages of Development

Although there is considerable variation in the age of onset of each stage, it is possible to identify general stages of phonological development and to relate them to the broader picture of language acquisition. The stages are:

1. **Prelinguistic stage (0;1–1;0)**   During the first year, the infant produces both speech-like and nonspeech-like vocalizations, with the former becoming predominant by the end of this stage. Although the speech-like vocalizations, or "babbling," have some of the sounds and timing characteristics of adult speech, they are considered "prelinguistic" because they lack the stable sound-meaning relationship that characterizes conventional words. From around 9 months, infants begin to demonstrate comprehension of words and simple phrases, and by 13 months the words in a child's receptive vocabulary number around 50 (Benedict, 1979).

2. **First words (1;0–1;6)**   This period is characterized by the onset of meaningful speech and the growth of productive vocabulary to about 50 words. There is, at this stage, considerable variation in the age of onset of meaningful speech and in the subsequent rate of lexical acquisition; Nelson (1973) found that some children had mastered 50 words by 14 months, whereas others did not have a 50-word vocabulary until they were 2;0. Phonologically, this period is characterized by productions of simple syllabic structure, typically CV (consonant–vowel), CVC, or CVCV. The repertoire of sound segments is relatively limited, consisting primarily of stops, nasals, and glides. The child's words seem to be learned and produced as *whole units* rather than as sequences of segments, and the first contrasts of the child's system are in terms of words; only later, during the next stage, is there evidence of contrasts in terms of phonemic oppositions (Ferguson, 1978). Because of the "whole-word" approach to word production and the concomitant lack of one-to-one correspondence between the phonemes of the adult word and those of the child's form, the first words are often understood only by the immediate family members who are familiar with the child's productive vocabulary and idiosyncratic way of pronouncing certain words. The end of this stage is signaled by a rapid increase in vocabulary size and by the onset of two-word utterances.

3. **Phonemic development (1;6–4;0)**   The vocabulary increase that occurs around 1;6 is accompanied by a marked change in the child's phonological system. The "whole-word" approach of the previous stage is no longer tenable once the vocabulary has grown to about 50 words and the child begins to produce rule-governed forms that have relatively stable segmental cor-

respondences with adult words. The number of different sound types increases, and the syllabic structures become more complex with the appearance of multisyllabic productions and consonant clusters. Some substitution patterns present during this period characterize the speech of most (perhaps all) children and are viewed by adults as typical of children's speech, e.g., [w] substituted for /r/, [f] for /θ/. Although the adult phonemic system is not fully acquired by the end of this stage, most phonemic contrasts are produced correctly at least some of the time by the typical 4-year-old (Sander, 1972). Syntactic and semantic development is also significant during this period, with the mean length of utterance rising from 1.2 to around 5.0 (Miller and Chapman, 1981).

4. **Stabilization of the phonological system (4;0–8;0)** During this stage, children stabilize their pronunciation of those phonemes that had been produced variably and acquire the last phonemes needed for completion of the phonetic inventory. Once in school, at around age 6;0, they are introduced to two important skills, reading and writing, that provide them with a conscious understanding of the phonemic nature of the sound system. They learn, for example, that a word can be broken up into discrete sound segments and represented in written form by a sequence of alphabetic symbols.

The various stages outlined above are described in greater detail in the following section.

Prelinguistic Stage

During the first year of life infants produce a variety of vocalizations ranging from cries and fussing to long sequences of consonant–vowel syllables with adult-like timing and intonation patterns. The productions can be divided into two general categories: (1) *reflexive* vocalizations (e.g., cries, coughs, and hiccups), which seem to be automatic responses reflecting the physical state of the infant; and (2) *nonreflexive* vocalizations (e.g., cooing, babbling, and playful yelling and screaming), which are nonautomatic productions containing some of the phonetic features found in adult languages (Oller, 1980; Stark, 1978).

All infants, regardless of the linguistic community in which they are being raised, seem to pass through the same stages of vocal development. The stages proposed by Oller (1980), with the approximate ages for each, are briefly described below. Although called "stages," the periods described are not discrete, and vocalizations typically overlap from one stage to another. However, each new stage is characterized by vocal behaviors not observed in the preceding period.

Stage 1 (0;0–0;1) This stage is characterized by a majority of reflexive vocalizations, e.g., crying, fussing, coughing, or burping. In addition, some nonreflexive sounds occur that are usually described as vowels or syllabic consonants.

Stage 2 (0;2–0;3) Often called the "cooing" or "gooing" stage, this stage is characterized by productions that are acoustically similar to back vowels or to syllables consisting of back consonants (velars, uvulars) and back vowels (Irwin, 1947; Zlatin, 1974). Oller (1980) cautioned that the CV syllables produced at this stage should be considered "primitive" because the timing of opening and closure of the consonantal and vocalic elements is far less regular than that which occurs in adult speech.

Stage 3 (0;4–0;6) This is a period of vocal play during which the infant seems to delight in exploring the capabilities of the vocal tract (Zlatin, 1974). Productions range from repetitions of vowel-like elements to squeals, growls, yells, raspberries (bilabial or labiolingual trills), and friction noises. The predominant type of vocalization can vary from week to week or even from day to day, making it difficult to characterize an infant's productions without an extensive sample. During this stage the infant produces some sequences of CV syllables; as in the previous stage, the timing of the opening and closure of these CV syllables is slow and irregular (Oller, 1980).

Stage 4 (0;7–0;9) This stage is characterized by vocalizations that are longer and consist of CV syllables whose timing approximates that of adult speech. The striking characteristic of the productions at this stage is the presence of reduplicated CV syllables, e.g., [mamama], [dadada] (Gesell and Armatruda, 1941; Nakazima, 1962; Smith and Oller, 1981). Upon hearing a sequence such as [mama] or [dada], parents often report with delight that their 7-month-old has begun to call them by name. At this stage, however, there is no evidence of a sound–meaning correspondence in the infant's productions, and thus [mama] cannot be considered a word. During this stage the repertoire of phones is relatively limited, with stops, nasals, and glides the most common consonantal sounds, and lax vowels, e.g., [ɛ, ɪ, ʌ], the most frequent vocalic types. The *place* of articulation of the consonantal phones shifts dramatically at about this stage as the frequency of velars declines sharply, whereas alveolars become predominant; labial consonants increase in frequency but do not supersede alveolars (Smith and Oller, 1981).

Stage 5 (0;10–1;0) This is a period of "variegated" babbling in which the productions are primarily CV sequences, as in the previous stage, but now the reduplicative nature of the utterances is no longer present and a variety of consonants and vowels can co-occur, e.g., [bawidu]. The consonantal repertoire also increases substantially during this period. A second characteristic of this stage is the presence of adult-like intonation patterns. Parents often believe their children are producing whole sentences—statements, questions, exclamations—but in their "own" language.

Locke (1983b) examined the results of more than a dozen babbling studies and found that although there was a fairly wide range of consonants produced during this stage their distribution varied dramatically. Data from three studies of English-learning infants ages 0;11–1;0 revealed that a set of 12 phones accounted for 92–97% of the consonants, whereas another 12 phones accounted for only 3–6% of the consonantal sounds. The frequently occurring sounds included primarily stops, nasals, and glides—[p,b,t,d,k,g,m,n,w,j,h,s]—whereas the infrequent sounds were mostly fricatives (except [s]), affricates, and liquids: [f,v,θ,ð,z,ʃ,ʒ,tʃ,ʤ,l,r,ŋ]. Thus although the *variety* of sounds increases during this stage, it must be kept in mind that certain sound classes occur with much greater frequency than other classes.

The prelinguistic stages outlined above seem for the most part to be maturationally determined. Infants from diverse linguistic communities and different socioeconomic backgrounds progress through the same stages at approximately the same ages. Even infants with linguistic handicaps, e.g., Down's syndrome, and hearing loss adhere to the same developmental schedule (Locke, 1983b). The earliest stages are influenced by changes in the form and size of the vocal tract. In newborn babies the tract resembles that of a nonhuman primate in that the tongue is large in relation to the oral cavity, the larynx is high in the neck, and because of the slope of the dorsal wall of the pharynx the posterior part of the tongue has little space in which to move (Kent, 1981; Lieber-man, 1971). Between 4 and 6 months there is a set of changes that allow the infant to produce a wider variety of sound types: (1) there is an increased separation of oral and nasal cavities; (2) the shape of the oral cavity changes with the appearance of teeth; and (3) the tongue becomes more mobile. The phonetic repertoire begins to expand at around 6 months, with the greatest increase occurring around 9–10 months.

Relationship Between Babbling and Speech

For many years the relationship between babbling and meaningful speech was viewed in one of two ways: (1) proponents of "babbling drift" (Brown, 1958; Mowrer, 1952) claimed that the prelinguistic vocalizations that most resembled adult speech were selectively reinforced by the infant's caretaker(s) and were gradually shaped so that they conformed with phonological patterns of the ambient language; and (2) the "discontinuity" theory (Jakobson, 1968) postulated that babbling and speech were two distinct stages of linguistic development that had little or no relationship to each other. The prelinguistic stage was said to be a period of vocal play characterized by "an astonishing quantity and diversity of sound productions," whereas the onset of meaningful speech was accompanied by the sudden *loss* of ability to produce a wide variety of sounds and by the slow (re)acquisition of phonemes for use in "true speech."

It is now obvious that neither of these views is tenable. If the *babbling drift* theory were true, we would find that the prelinguistic vocalizations of infants raised in Chinese-, Spanish-, and English-speaking environments, for example, would differ markedly by the end of the first year. The Chinese-learning baby would produce utterances that, although not replications of adult words, would resemble Chinese in terms of sound segments, syllable structures, and intonational patterns; in like fashion, the utterances of the babies raised in the other linguistic communities would share the phonological patterns of the ambient language. To date, there is no evidence to support this view. Studies have shown that adults, even trained phoneticians, cannot perceive differences between the babbling of babies from different linguistic environments even at the end of the prelinguistic period when the influence of the ambient language would presumably be the strongest (Atkinson et al., 1968; Olney and Scholnick, 1976), and that neither acoustic analyses (Eady, 1980) nor phonetic transcriptions of the segmental and syllabic types (Locke, 1983b) reveal differences between these babies.

The *discontinuity* view has also received little support from the existing data. Jakobson (1968) stated that there was often a period of silence marking the end of the babbling stage and the beginning of "true words," and that there were marked differences in the phonetic repertoires of the two periods. Although there is individual variation in the amount of overlap between the two stages, it seems that most children continue to babble for at least 3–4 months after the appearance of their first words. In addition, the results of studies covering the transition from babbling to speech reveal that the phonological patterns of babbling are quite similar to those of early meaningful speech in terms of syllabic types and phonetic repertoires (Stoel-Gammon and Cooper, 1981; Vihman et al., 1981); these findings do not support Jakobson's contention that babbling and speech represent two unrelated stages of linguistic development with little in common.

Transition to Speech

The child does not simply stop babbling one day and begin to speak the next. Rather, there is a period of overlap, lasting from a few weeks to several months, during which babbled utterances and meaningful speech co-occur. In some instances, real words are embedded in babbled phrases (Branigan, 1977). Description and classification of vocalizations produced during this period are further complicated by the presence of proto-words (or vocables), which have *some* phonetic and semantic consistency and thus cannot be categorized as babbling but do not have the stable sound–meaning relationships characteristic of adult words. According to Ferguson (1978), a child's early vocabulary "typically consists of a dozen or so vocables of which only one or two are apparently based on adult words; most of the rest are apparently based on nonspeech noise or a babbling sound originally uttered by the child in a certain context and used by him when the context recurs, or when he wants to allude to it."

Halliday (1975) traced the early linguistic development of his son Nigel, providing a detailed account of the proto-words, their meaning, and their function. Some examples, produced around Nigel's first birthday, are shown below:

Gloss	Phonetic form (tone)
Yes I want that	[yiyiyi] (high level)
Do that (again)	[a] (mid)
Look, a picture; you say what it is	[a::da] (high rise and mid fall)
Let's pretend to go to sleep	[gʷɤɪ (2–4x)] (narrow low)
That tastes nice	[ʔn̥ŋ] (low)
That's nice	[ɛʸ] or [i:] (low)

It is clear from these examples that the phonetic forms Nigel was producing were not directly modeled on an adult word but were invented, as it were, by the child. (See Dore, 1976, for further examples.) In some cases, however, words that start out as invented forms develop into regular vocabulary clearly linked to adult words in both sound and meaning. In a study of a single subject (David), Carter (1974, 1979) followed the development of these forms from "sensori-motor morphemes," as she called them, to real words. Between ages 1;1 and 1;2, David produced forms that differed from babbling in two ways: they had some phonetic consistency, and their production was regularly accompanied by a specific gesture. For example, David said [mm], [ma], [may], or [mə] as he reached for an object; [la], [læ], [da], [dæ], or [də] as he pointed at an object; and [hɪ], [hɪy], [he], [hə], or [hm] as he was giving or receiving an object. Carter believed that these gesture-accompanying sounds serve as the basis for the subsequent acquisition of the conventional words shown below.

Vocable	Gesture	Conventional words
m + V (V = vowel)	Reaching for an object	More, my, mine
l + V, d + V	Pointing at an object	Look, these, this, the, that, there
h + V	Giving or receiving an object	Here, where, have

Although Ferguson (1978) claimed that children typically have nearly a dozen vocables in the early stages of language development, subsequent research has not supported his claim. It seems that most, perhaps all, children include some vocables in their early vocabulary but that the number of such forms varies extensively. In a study of three children, Stoel-Gammon and Cooper (1981) reported that one child used 13 vocables during the period of acquiring 50 conventional (i.e., adult-based) words. In contrast, the other two subjects had only one vocable each during the same period. None of the children produced vocables that subsequently developed into adult-based words, as was the case with Carter's subject (1974, 1979). More research is needed to fully document the frequency and use of these forms in early speech.

First "Real" Words

At the same time the child is producing proto-words, he or she is also attempting to pronounce words based on an adult model. In many instances the child's form is very different from the adult's making it difficult to identify without help from the linguistic and situational context. Studies of the phonetic form of these words have revealed common patterns in their overall form and in the sounds that occur (Jakobson, 1968; Stoel-Gammon, 1984; Winitz and Irwin, 1958). According to these studies, the child's words are most commonly a single syllable, or fully or partially reduplicated syllables, e.g., [baba] or [mami]; closed syllables (CVC as opposed to CV) also occur but less frequently. In terms of *manner* of production, the consonantal sounds are primarily stops, nasals, or glides, the same sound types that predominated during the late babbling period; fricatives occur less frequently and vary considerably from child to child. Regarding *place* of articulation, labial and alveolar consonants tend to be frequent, whereas palatals and velars are less common.

Table 2.1 presents the first 35 conventional words of three children: Daniel, Sarah, and Will (Stoel-Gammon and Cooper, 1981). The words are listed in approximate order of acquisition, and phonetic variations are shown for words with unstable pronunciations. The table provides a good illustration of the similarities and differences found in the early stages of meaningful speech. Examination of the consonantal phones in the children's productions shows that the words are composed primarily, but not exclusively, of stops and nasals. The chart below presents the consonantal phones produced by each child; to be included in the chart, each phone had to occur in at least *two* words in the child's vocabulary:

	Daniel	Sarah	Will
Stops	t k ʔ	t k	pw t ʔ
	b d g	b d	b d g
Fric/affric	s ʒ	ʃ	s ts z
Nasals	n	m n	m
Glides	w	w h	
Liquids		l	

Table 2.1 First 35 Words in Three Children Ages 0;11–1;5

Daniel		Sarah		Will	
Gloss	Transcription	Gloss	Transcription	Gloss	Transcription
light	daɪ, aɪ	baby	bebi	uh-oh	ʔʌʔo, hʌho
uh-oh	ʌʔoʔ	mommy	mama	all-done	ada, dada
what's that	wɜsæʔ	doggie	dɔgi	light	di
wow	waʊ	juice	dus	down	dæ, dʌ, daʊ
banana	nænə	bye-bye	baɪbaɪ	shoes	tʃɪs, θɪz
kitty	kiː, kɪdi	daddy	dædæ	baby	didi
baby	didi, titi	milk	ma	don't throw	dõtwo, dõpwo
moo	mu, mbu	cracker	kækæ	moo	βu
quack	gak	done	dʌ̃n, dʌ̃	bite	bʌ, ba
cookie	koki	ball	ba	three	pwi, bwi
nice	naɪ	shoe	ʃ̩	hi	aɪ
rock	gak, ak	teddy	dɛɪ̯, tɛɪ̯	cheese	ti, tiz, tʃi
clock	gak, ak	book	bi	up	ʌʔ, ʌʔʌʔ
sock	gak	kitty	kiki, titi	quack-quack	gægæ
woof-woof	βuβu, uɸuɸ	hi	haɪ	oink-oink	gægæ
daddy	dædi, dæi	Allie	æli	coat	go, gogo
bubble	bʌbu	no	no	beep-beep	bibi

hi	aɪ	door	dowə	keys	dɪz, dɪs
shoe	ʒ;, ʒə, əʒ	dolly	dɔli	cycle	gɪgə
up	ʌp, bʌp	what's that	wʌdæ	mama	mama
bye-bye	daɪdaɪ	cheese	tʃiʃ	daddy	dæi, dædæ
bottle	babu	oh wow	owaʊ	siren sound	ĩ
no	no	oh	o:	grr	gu
rocky	gaki, aki	button	bi, bʌdi	more	mʌ, ma
eye	aɪ	eye	aɪ	off	ɔ
nose	no	apple	æfpl̩	tick-tock	tɪta
fire	aɪ	nose	nõ, no	ball	ba, bʌ, bɔ
hot	atʃ, at	bird	bɪ	go	go, do
yogurt	gogu, ogu	all-done	ada	bump	bʌ
pee-pee	didi, titi	orange	owɪʒ, owi	pop-pop	baba
juice	ʒus, zus	bottle	babi	out	ʊ
ball	ba	coat	dot, do	hee-haw	iʔa
whack	gak, ak	hot	ha	eat	i:
frog	gak	bib	bɪə	neigh	ne, nene
hello	ɛwo, o	hat	hæ	meow	ija

From Stoel-Gammon and Cooper, 1981.

25

The number of phones in each child's inventory is the same—10 for each. Moreover, the manner of production of the phones was highly similar, with stops predominating in all cases. The children's productions are alike not only in terms of consonantal sounds but also syllabic structure. For Sarah and Will, the most frequent syllable shapes were CV and CVCV, where the two consonants were often the same. For Daniel, the syllable shapes were more varied—CV, CVCV, VC, CVC—with no single type predominating.

Despite the general similarities in children's early words, analysis of the data on an individual levels reveals considerable variation. One important individual difference lies in the adult words children choose to include in their vocabularies. For many years it was believed that words were included in a child's vocabulary because of their semantic and grammatical properties (Nelson, 1973); children used words that allowed them to: (1) name objects or persons of interest: *kitty, ball, Mommy*; (2) describe or demand an action: *give, bye-bye, up*; and (3) interact socially: *thank you, no, yes*. Now there is evidence that phonological characteristics of the adult word also play an important role in determining which words will be included in the early vocabulary. A number of studies (Ferguson and Farwell, 1975; Menn, 1976b; Schwartz and Leonard, 1982; Vihman, 1981) have shown patterns of lexical selection based on phonological characteristics of the adult words.

The specific word selection patterns vary widely from child to child, but generally seem to be based on the syllabic structure and/or sound segments of the adult word. For example, the first five words of Jonathan Braine were all adult monosyllables of the form CV or CVC: *hi, there/that, no, juice, see* (Braine, 1974), whereas Leslie, a child studied by Ferguson et al. (1973), chose CVCV forms ending in [i]: *mommy, daddy, doggie, patty* (from pat-a-cake). In terms of sound segments or classes of sounds, Ferguson and Farwell (1975) presented data from "T," whose first 50 words contained 15 beginning with a labial and 10 that contained a fricative, usually a sibilant, as the initial or final element.

If we look at the data for Daniel, Sarah, and Will (Table 2.1), word selection patterns can be identified for Daniel and Will but not for Sarah. Daniel seems to prefer words with a particular sound type, velar stops, particularly /k/; 10 of his 35 words contain at least one velar stop. Will's early vocabulary includes a high proportion of two types of words: (1) forms that are fully or partially reduplicated, e.g., *quack-quack, mama, tick-tock*; and (2) onomatopoeic forms, e.g., *moo, grr, beep-beep, meow*.

Selection patterns that show a *preference* for words with specific phonological characteristics are fairly easy to document, whereas patterns showing an *avoidance* of certain sounds or syllable types are more difficult as it is almost impossible to know if a child fails to produce something by choice or by chance. A fairly convincing example of avoidance is described by Menn (1976b) in her detailed study of Jacob. Unlike most children, whose early vocabularies include some labial-initial words (typically *baby* and *bottle* among others), Jacob attempted no words beginning with /p/ or /b/ for several months. Until he was 19 months old his only *b*-initial word was *bye-bye;* then he added *box* to his vocabulary followed shortly by five other words beginning with /b/. Although he had adopted some *b*-initial words, Jacob had no words beginning with /p/ until he was 20 months old. The lack of labial-initial words in Menn's subject is particularly apparent when his vocabulary is compared with other children at the same stage of development. Each of the vocabularies shown in Table 2.1, for example, contains at least a half-dozen words which, in the adult form, begin with a labial stop.

When children's selection and avoidance patterns are compared with their production patterns, it seems that they select words with phonological characteristics that are consistent with their developing phonological systems and avoid words with characteristics outside their system. Thus the child "T" (Ferguson and Farwell, 1975), whose vocabulary included a high proportion of words with initial labial stops, accurately produced the voicing distinction between /p/ and /b/ at around age 1;1. For most children, correct production is not attained for another 12–18 months (Macken and Barton, 1980). Likewise, Daniel (Table 2.1) chose adult words with velar stops and produced those stops accurately, whereas Jacob (Menn, 1976b), who avoided words with initial labials, seemed to have difficulty pronouncing [p-] and [b-]. *Bye-bye,* his only labial-initial word until he was 19 months old, was produced with [d] rather than [b].

The notion of selection and avoidance patterns was formally tested by Schwartz and Leonard (1982) in an experimental setting. They presented young children with nonsense words such as /kɪt/ to denote "actions that spin objects" and /ofof/ for "object at the end of a string or chain" and found that imitation and spontaneous production of these words was more likely to occur if the syllabic structures and consonantal phonemes of the nonsense words occurred in the subject's own productions. That is, the children tended to *select* words with sounds and syllable shapes they could produce and *avoid* words with sounds and syllabic structures outside their repertoire. These findings seem to support the hypothesis that lexical acquisition is based, at least in part, on phonological characteristics of the adult word and production patterns of the child.

As in other aspects of phonological development, there is much individual variation in selection patterns and how they relate to production. Some children are quite conservative, choosing words they can produce accurately. For others, accuracy does not seem to be so important; rather, they are quite willing to restructure the adult word so that it will fit into an articulation pattern they are capable of producing. For example, Jonathan Braine (Braine, 1974), whose first five words were adult monosyllables of the form CV or CVC, used the articulation pattern [dV] (V is a vowel) for pronouncing four of the five words; *see* [di], *no* [do], *juice* [du], *that/there* [dʌ], [dɛ], or [dæ]. Subsequent additions to his vocabulary also conformed to this pattern: *pee* [di], *car* [da], *door* [dɔ]. Of these early productions, the initial consonant of Jonathan's form and the adult form matched in only one word: *door*.

Daniel (cited in Table 2.1) showed a preference for adult words with velar stops. He also had a basic production pattern for pronouncing these words; the pattern CVC or CVCV, where both consonants (C) were velar stops, was used in the pronunciation of *quack, cookie, rock, clock, sock, yogurt, rocky, frog, whack, yuk, block,* and *milk* at around age 1;4 (Stoel-Gammon and Cooper, 1981). Such a production pattern created many homophones in Daniel's output, with *quack, rock, clock, sock, frog, yuk, block,* and *milk* all pronounced [gak].

Summary

The first word stage is difficult to summarize succinctly because of the extensive individual differences that have been documented. Although there are similarities across children in terms of the sound segment and syllabic types produced, there are at the same time differences in the adult words attempted and in the production patterns used in their pronunciation. These differences relate to patterns of preference for, and avoidance of, particular sounds or sound classes or certain syllabic shapes and have been observed by a number of researchers (e.g., Ferguson and Farwell, 1975; Ferguson et al., 1973; Menn, 1976b; Vihman, 1981). However, at least one study has shown that such patterns do not appear in the speech of *all* children (Stoel-Gammon and Cooper, 1981). Given the small number of subjects involved in most of the research (usually one to three children), no conclusive statements regarding the frequency of these patterns can be made. On the one hand, they may be universal or near-universal; on the other, they may be relatively infrequent. Additional research focusing on this aspect of early development will provide the answers.

Developing a System

The end of the first-word stage is marked in two ways. First, there is a rapid increase in vocabulary size and a relaxation of selection constraints on adult words the child attempts to produce (Schwartz and Leonard, 1982). Second, the relationship between the sounds of the adult model and the child's pronunciation becomes more systematic. During the period of the first words, whole words (rather than phonemes) seem to be the basic unit of contrast. According to Ferguson (1978), "the child remembers and recognizes the phonetic shapes of whole words and articulates in terms of phonetic word-shapes." (This notion of words as unanalyzed phonetic units has a parallel in early syntactic development, where the child produces word combinations such as *have-it* or *it's-a* as single words, e.g., I *have-it* blue car. *It's-a* falling down.)

As mentioned in the previous chapter, early productions cannot be adequately described in terms of phonemes because the unit "phoneme" implies a stable behavior within and across lexical items. In addition, the relationship between the child's pronunciation of a word and the adult model cannot be described in terms of phonological rules because rules are based on systematic correspondences between the two forms. When the vocabulary begins to expand rapidly, typically around age 1;6–1;10, the child's productions become more stable and systematic correspondences between the adult and child form emerge. It has been argued that rapid vocabulary growth forces the child to adopt a rule-governed approach to his phonological productions, resulting in a system based primarily on phonemes, rather than whole words (Ingram, 1976; Menn, 1979).

Once a rule-based system appears, phonological development proceeds rapidly, and by age 4;0 the average English-speaking child can produce a majority of sounds correctly (Sander, 1972). Our knowledge of phonological acquisition during this period comes from two types of investigation: formal studies involving large numbers of subjects at varying ages and longitudinal studies of a single child or a small group of children (typically not more than eight).

Large-scale studies serve as a basis for determining normative stages of phonological development; the results provide information regarding age of mastery and error types. Longitudinal studies provide detailed accounts of development and, when grouped together, allow us to determine something about the range of individual differences that may occur. Although each type of investigation has certain weaknesses (discussed in detail in Chapter 4), both provide valuable information to the field of child phonology. In the discussion of segmental acquisition that follows, the findings of the large-scale studies are presented first, followed by a brief discussion of longitudinal studies of individual or small groups of children.

Segmental Acquisition

Single Phonemes Investigations of large groups of children, like those of Prather et al. (1975), Poole (1934), Templin (1957), and Wellman et al. (1931), focused on the age of mastery of the phonemes of English. Consonantal phonemes were usually tested in initial, medial, and final position and were said to be "mastered" when a certain percentage (75% in most cases) of the subjects at a given age produced them correctly in all positions tested. Although there were some age differences across the studies (due primarily to methodological differences in the data collection and analysis), the order of acquisition of sounds and sound classes was remarkably similar: stops, nasals, and glides are mastered first, then liquids, and finally fricatives and affricates. Templin's findings, shown in Table 2.2, illustrate the general pattern of acquisition.

Table 2.2 Age of Mastery[a]
of Consonantal Phonemes

Age	Phoneme
3;0	p, m, n, ŋ, f, w
3;6[b]	j
4;0	b, k, g, r
4;6	s, ʃ, tʃ
5;0	
6;0	t, l, θ, v
7;0	ð, z, ʒ, ʤ

Adapted from Templin (1957).

[a]A phoneme is "mastered" when produced correctly by 75% of the subjects.

[b]The phonemes are listed cumulatively by age; only newly mastered phonemes are shown for each age.

Sander (1972) reviewed the data from the studies of Wellman (1931), Poole (1934), and Templin (1957) and suggested that the findings would be more useful if they were presented in two ways, showing both the age of *customary production* (defined as the age level at which "the combined test average at the various word positions exceeds 50% correct production") and the age of *mastery* (defined as the age level at which "the combined test average reaches 90% correct production") (Sander, 1972). His reanalysis of Templin's (1957) and Wellman et al.'s (1931) data along these lines is presented in Table 2.3. It is clear from this reanalysis that the time span between the age of customary production of sounds and age of mastery is greater for fricatives and affricates than for other sound classes, ranging up to 5 years for the phoneme /s/.

Although the results of the large-scale studies suggest that there are universal or near-universal patterns of order of acquisition of consonantal phonemes, longitudinal investigations reveal considerable variation in the order. For example, Macken (1980a) examined diary accounts of five children learning English and found no consistent order of acquisition of stop consonants in terms of place of production. Edwards (1978, 1979) analyzed longitudinal data from six children (ages approximately 1;6–2;6) and concluded that: "There is no universal order of acquisition for fricatives" (Edwards, 1979).

The discrepancy between the two types of study is due primarily to differences in data collection and analysis. The large-scale studies report children's performances at 6-month or yearly inter-

Table 2.3 Age of Customary Production and Mastery of Consonantal Phonemes

Age	Consonants Customarily Produced	Consonants Mastered
Before 2;0	p, b, m, n, w, hᵃ	
2;0ᵇ	t, d, k, g, ŋ	
3;0	f, s, r, l, j	p, m, n, w, h
4;0	v, z, ʃ, tʃ, ʤ	b, d, k, g, f, j
5;0	θ, ð	
6;0	ʒᶜ	t, ŋ, r, l
7;0		θ, ʃ, tʃ, ʤ
8;0		v, ð, s, ʒ

Adapted from Sander (1972).

ᵃThese consonants exceeded 70% correct production at 2;0, the youngest level tested.

ᵇThe phonemes are listed cumulatively; only new phonemes are shown for each age.

ᶜThis consonant was not "mastered" by 8;0 and thus does not appear in the right-hand column.

vals, whereas the longitudinal studies describe acquisition on a daily or weekly basis. If a child is tested at yearly intervals and acquires the phonemes /t, d, k, g/ between the ages of 2;0 and 3;0, there is no way of knowing the exact order of acquisition of the four phonemes. Only if data collection occurs more frequently will that information be available.

Word Position When Templin's (1957) data are presented by *position* of the target sound within the word, as in Table 2.4, it is apparent that some consonants (e.g., /p, s, θ/ are acquired in all three positions at a single age level, whereas others (e.g., /t, l, ʤ/ are acquired first in one or two positions but much later in another position. In general, consonants in final position, particularly voiced stops, are shown to be mastered later than consonants in other positions.

Some investigations of children younger than those studied by Templin have suggested that fricatives (Farwell, 1977; Ferguson, 1975) and velars (Ingram, 1974) may appear first in final position. However, these findings were not supported by Stoel-Gammon's longitudinal study (1984) of 34 children ages 1;3–2;0. Her study did reveal one consistent difference between initial and final position: the phoneme /r/ appeared word finally well before it oc-

Table 2.4 Age of Mastery[a] of Consonantal Phonemes by Initial, Medial, and Final Position

			Manner Class		
Age	Nasal	Stop	Liquid, Glide	Fricative	Affricate
3;0	m, n, ŋ	p, b-,[b] -b- t-, -t, d-, -d- k-, -k-, g-, -g-	w, h, j -r	f	
4;0[c]		-b, -d, -k, -g	l-, -l- r-, -r-	s, ʃ -z-, -v-	tʃ ʤ-
5;0					-ʤ-
6;0		-t-	-l	θ, ð- v-, -v	
7;0				-ð-, -ð z-, -z ʒ	-ʤ

Adapted from Templin (1957).

[a]A phoneme is "mastered" when produced correctly by 75% of the subjects.

[b]A dash indicates position in the word; if the phoneme is not shown with a dash, it was mastered in all three positions.

[c]The phonemes are listed cumulatively; only newly mastered phonemes are shown for each age.

curred word initially. In conclusion, it should be noted that there is substantial individual variation regarding the effect of word position on phonemic acquisition. Kiparsky and Menn (1977), for example, described a child who produced all new phones first in final position.

Consonant Clusters Templin's study included norms on the mastery of consonant clusters as well as single segments. Her findings, presented in Table 2.5, show that by the age of 4;0, 75% of the subjects correctly produced initial clusters composed of /s + stop/, /s + nasal/, /stop + liquid/ (except /gr/), and /stop + w/. Fewer final clusters are acquired by age 4;0, and the pattern of acquisition in terms of sound classes is not as regular. In general, final nasal clusters (except those with /n/) are acquired by 4;0 and liquid + stop clusters by 6;0; liquid + fricative and fricative + stop, however, are not mastered until 7;0.

Longitudinal studies (e.g., Greenlee, 1973, 1974; Moskowitz, 1971) revealed substantial differences in rate and order of acquisition of clusters and in the types of errors. These differences make it difficult to identify developmental stages between the first attempts at production and final mastery. We clearly need further research in this area before definitive statements can be made.

Table 2.5 Age of Mastery[a] of Consonant Clusters

Age	Initial Clusters	Final Clusters
4;0	pl, bl, kl, gl pr, br, tr, dr, kr tw, kw sm, sn, sp, st, sk	mp, mpt, mps, ŋk lp, lt, rm, rt, rk pt, ks ft
5;0[b]	gr, fl, fr, str	lb, lf rd, rf, rn
6;0	skw	lk rb, rg, rθ, rdʒ, rst, rtʃ nt, nd, nθ
7;0	spl, spr, skr sl, sw ʃr, θr	sk, st, kst lθ, lz dʒd
8;0		kt, sp

Adapted from Templin (1957).

[a]A cluster is "mastered" when produced correctly by 75% of the subjects.

[b]The clusters are listed cumulatively; only newly mastered clusters are listed for each age.

Suprasegmental Development

The term *suprasegmental* refers to prosodic features, e.g., rhythm, intonation, and stress, that can be superimposed over a sequence of sound segments. Physical attributes of the speech signal, e.g., fundamental frequency, intensity, and timing, serve as cues for the perception of prosodic features but cannot be directly equated with any given feature. Although suprasegmentals play an important role in the production and perception of speech, relatively little research has been done on their development in children. Our knowledge in this area is summarized below.

Intonation Intonation, defined as "the perceived patterned rise and fall of pitch over linguistic units" (Freeman, 1982), is related most closely to the acoustic property of fundamental frequency. In English, intonational contours are used to mark utterance boundaries and to distinguish between certain types of sentences, e.g., statement versus question versus exclamation. Adult-like intonational contours have been reported as appearing early in infant vocal productions and can be imitated by infants as young as 4 months old (Kuhl and Meltzoff, 1982). By 9–10 months, children use rising and falling contours in such a way that parents often believe that their children are asking questions and making statements in their "own language." Intonational patterns are present at all stages of meaningful speech, even in the one-word stage. Careful study of their use, however, reveals that the rising and falling patterns do not seem to be based on adult sentence patterns of rising contours for questions and falling ones for statements (Miller and Ervin, 1964). In fact, some children have been reported to develop quite idiosyncratic patterns of intonation (Bloom, 1973; Halliday, 1975).

Stress and Rhythm The suprasegmental feature *stress* involves several parameters, including pitch, duration, and loudness. Stressed syllables are perceived as higher pitched, longer, and louder than unstressed syllables. Prosodic *rhythm*, defined as "the perception of a patterned time program underlying sequences of speech" (Freeman, 1982), is closely related to stress. In a "stress-timed" language such as English (i.e., a language in which the stressed syllables are perceived as being evenly spaced), the rhythmic pattern is based on an alternating arrangement of stressed and unstressed syllables.

Studies of the development of stress and rhythm indicate that young children have difficulty producing *unstressed* rather than stressed syllables (Allen, 1976; Allen and Hawkins, 1980). Unstressed syllables are often deleted; when produced, they are often articulated with less accuracy than stressed syllables of comparable phonetic complexity. Klein (1981) presented data from two young children who had distinctly different patterns for producing words with unstressed syllables. One child tended to delete the syllable, e.g., *giraffe* (wæf), *needle* [niə], *butterfly* [baɪɸaɪ], while the second child produced the syllable but assimilated it to a stressed syllable, e.g., *bunny* ['babi], *bulldozer* ['budədə], *alligator* ['ægigi].

Gleitman and Wanner (1982) pointed out that the feature *stress* plays an important role in syntactic and morphological as well as phonological development. They noted that the phenomenon of "telegraphic speech" (Brown and Bellugi, 1964) and the differences observed in the acquisition of inflectional affixes across languages, e.g., early in Turkish, late in Russian (Slobin, 1982), can be explained by the fact that stressed items are acquired early whereas unstressed items are often omitted in the initial stages.

Timing There are two major aspects of speech timing that distinguish between child and adult speech: rate and variability. On the whole, children speak more slowly than adults and do not achieve adult-like rates of production until they are 11–12 years old (Kent, 1976). Smith (1978) analyzed word and segment durations of nonsense words and found that word durations were 31% longer for 2-year-olds than for adults and 15% longer for 4-year-olds than for adults. His measurements of segment durations revealed that, on the average, segments produced by 2-year-olds were 50 ms longer than those produced by adults; for 4-year-olds, the average increase was 25 ms per segment in comparison with the adult values. In spite of the greater absolute values observed in the 2- and 4-year-olds, Smith noted that the proportional durations of the segments were similar for all three subject groups; for example, comparison of durations of stressed and unstressed vowels revealed that proportional values of the groups differed by no more than 3%.

Child speech is not only slower than adult speech, it is more variable. When a young child produces multiple repetitions of a word or utterance the segmental durations vary considerably, and the younger the child the greater the variability (Eguchi and Hirsch, 1969; Tingley and Allen, 1975). Variability in segment durations as well as in fundamental frequency and vowel formant frequencies decreases with age; by the time children are around 11;0–13;0, the variability in their speech is comparable to that reported for adult speech (Kent, 1976).

Incorrect Productions

Our knowledge of phonological development comes not only from analyses of what is produced but also from examining the types of errors that occur. Analyses of incorrect productions show that children's pronunciations are related to the adult forms in systematic ways. The relationship between the adult form and the child's pronunciation can be described in terms of phonetic features, phonemes, phonological rules based on distinctive features, or phonological processes. We have chosen to use *phonological processes* because we believe this approach provides the simplest and most economical way of describing the differences in the structural and segmental aspects of the two forms. The error patterns described here are based on findings of longitudinal case studies, investigations of small groups of children, and large-scale studies (e.g., Olmsted, 1971).

The notion of phonological processes was introduced by Stampe in 1969 (see also Stampe, 1973) and has been widely adopted in the field of child phonology (Ingram, 1976). According to Stampe (1969), a phonological process is a *mental operation* that "merges a potential phonological opposition into that member of the opposition which least tries the restrictions of the human speech capacity." It is clear from this definition that for Stampe, and presumably for other researchers who use them, phonological processes have some sort of psychological reality. We do not agree. Although we believe that phonological processes provide a useful framework for describing children's systematic simplifications of the adult phonological system, we do not ascribe to the view that they are psychologically real. The data currently available are simply not sufficient to allow us to determine the psychological status of pronunciation errors; thus, at present, phonological processes provide a means for *describing*, but not *explaining*, the error patterns evident in young children's speech. The most common error patterns are described in the sections that follow. They are grouped into three major categories: (1) processes that modify the syllabic structure of the target word; (2) processes that substitute one sound for another; and (3) processes that assimilate one sound to another. Nearly all the processes *simplify* the adult form in one way or another; in many cases the simplification results in loss of a phonemic contrast (see discussion of individual processes below). The description is limited to those processes that have been reported to occur commonly in the speech of young children.

Syllable Structure Processes Syllable structure processes are changes that modify the syllabic structures of the target word. These include:

1. **Unstressed Syllable Deletion (USD)** Deletion of an unstressed syllable or syllables:

tomato	medo	telephone	tɛfon
pajama	ʤæmə	about	baʊt
elephant	ɛfənt	beside	saɪd

   In some cases, segments from different syllables are coalesced into a single syllable:

pacifier	pæf	balloon	bun
garage	gaʒ	banana	bænə

2. **Final Consonant Deletion (FCD)** Deletion of a final consonant or consonant cluster:

dog	da	bean	bi
car	ka	mouse	maʊ
park	pa	milk	mɪ

   When Final Consonant Deletion occurs consistently, it can create homophonous forms that make a child's speech highly unintelligible. For example, the adult words *cap, cab, calf, cat,* and *can* are all pronounced [kæ], and *beep, beat, bead, beef, beach,* and *bean* are all [bi]. Before final consonants begin to appear, some children maintain the phonemic contrast of the adult form by accurately producing distinctive features of the vowel. For example, in words ending in a nasal consonant, e.g., *can* and *bean*, the vowel is nasalized: [kæ̃] and [bĩ]; in words ending in an obstruent, the voicing distinction is preserved by differences in vowel length, e.g., *cap* [kæ] versus *cab* [kæ:], *beat* [bi] versus *bead* [bi:], *bus* [bʌ] versus *buzz* [bʌ:]. Although the resultant productions are still incorrect, they preserve phonetic distinctions found in the adult form and thus may be easier to understand.

3. **Doubling (Dbl)** The repetition of a target word, usually a monosyllabic word, creating a multisyllabic form. This process is often accompanied by final consonant deletion, as shown in the production of *dog* and *ball* below:

go	gogo	walk	wakwak
dog	dada	ball	baba

(Other reduplicated forms are described under assimilation process.)

4. **Diminutization (Dim)**   Addition of [i], or sometimes [Ci] (C = consonant), to the target form:

cup	kʌpi	coat	kodi
egg	ɛgi	no	nodi

5. **Cluster Reduction (CR)**   Simplification of a consonant cluster by reducing it to one sound (or to two sounds if the target cluster consists of three consonants). The actual form of the reduction differs according to the type of target cluster; the most common reduction patterns are described below.

   a. In /stop + liquid/ clusters, the stop is usually maintained and the liquid deleted:

bread	bɛd	glass	gæs
drink	dɪŋk	blue	bu

   b. In post-vocalic clusters composed of /liquid + stop/ or /liquid + nasal/, the liquid is usually deleted:

dark	dak	milk	mɪk
bird	bʊd	cold	kod

   c. In /s + stop/ and /s + nasal/ clusters, /s/ is usually deleted:

skip	kɪp	snow	no
stop	tap	smoke	mok
ask	æk		

   Some children go through a stage in the production of /s + nasal/ clusters in which the /s/ is deleted and the nasal is produced as a voiceless segment. The child Amahl Smith (Smith, 1973), for example, produced *smell* as [mɛl] at one stage, later as [m̥ɛl] with a voiceless *m*; similarly, *snake* was [neik] and then [n̥eik]. The presence of a voiceless nasal serves to maintain a phonological distinction that would otherwise be lost; for example, when /sn/ is reduced to [n̥], the words *snow* [n̥o] and *no* [no] are pronounced differently.

   d. Clusters composed of /nasal + obstruent/ are usually reduced in one of two ways: if the obstruent is voiced, it is deleted; if the obstruent is voiceless, the nasal is deleted:

mend	mɛn	bump	bʌp
hand	hæn	ant	æt
candy	kæni	pinch	pɪtʃ

e. Whereas most clusters are reduced by deleting one member and maintaining the other, some initial clusters are reduced to a single sound that was *not* a member of the target cluster; commonly occurring examples are:

| truck | fʌk | swing | fɪŋ |
| tree | fi | sweep | fip |

6. **Epenthesis (Ep)** Insertion of an unstressed vowel, usually [ə]. This process usually occurs in one of two environments:

a. In the production of an initial cluster:

| blue | bəlu | sleep | səlip |
| green | gərin | swing | səwɪŋ |

b. After a final voiced stop:

| big | bɪgə | bib | bɪbə |
| bad | bædə | | |

Epenthetic vowels in final position seem to occur as the first stage of a voicing contrast between stops in word-final position. Thus *bead* may first be pronounced [bit], then [biːt] with vowel lengthening, then [biːdə], and finally [biːd].

Substitution Processes Substitution processes are those sound changes that substitute one class of sounds for another. The substitution processes are grouped according to the target phonemes they affect.

1. **Liquids**
   a. *Gliding (G)* Substitution of glide for a prevocalic liquid; /r/ is usually replaced by [w], /l/ by either [w] or [j]. In some children the substitution patterns for /l/ is determined by the following vowel: /l/ is substituted by [j] before front vowels, by [w] elsewhere. Examples of gliding include:

rabbit	wæbɪt	look	wʊk
ring	wɪŋ	balloon	bəwun
merry	mɛwi	leaf	jif

Gliding also occurs in consonant clusters:

| bread | bwɛd | blow | bwo |
| grass | gwæs | glass | gwæs |

b. *Vocalization (Voc)*   Substitution of a vowel, usually [o] or [u], for a syllabic liquid:

noodle	nudu	butter	bʌdu
bottle	badu	zipper	zɪpu
uncle	ʌŋku	hammer	hæmo

This substitution pattern may also affect postvocalic non-syllabic liquids:

fell	fɛu̯	deer	diu̯
cold	kou̯d	farm	fau̯m

2. Fricatives

a. *Stopping (S)*   Substitution of a stop for a fricative or affricate, or an affricate for a fricative. This process occurs most commonly in word-initial position, although it can occur in other positions as well. As shown in the examples, the general *place of articulation* of the target phoneme is maintained while the manner of articulation changes:

feet	pit, p̪fit	TV	tibi
vacuum	bækjum	house	haʊt
that	dæt	nose	nod
juice	dus	beach	bit

b. *Depalatalization (Dep):*   Substitution of an alveolar fricative for a palatal fricative, or an alveolar affricate for a palatal affricate:

ship	sɪp	chin	t̪sɪn
shoe	su	watch	wat̪s
fish	fɪs	jar	d̪zar

3. Stops and Nasals

a. *Velar Fronting (VF)*   Substitution of an alveolar for a velar consonant. This process occurs more commonly in initial than in final position.

key	ti	make	met
cow	taʊ	book	bʊt
go	do	bang	bæn

Assimilation Processes   Assimilation processes are sound changes in which one sound becomes more similar to another. Assimilations are classified as *progressive* if the sound which causes the assimilation precedes the affected sound, as *regressive* if it follows the affected sound. The most common types of assimilation are described below:

1. **Consonant harmony** (also called consonant assimilation)
   Noncontiguous assimilation of one consonant to another in
   terms of place or manner of production. Commonly occurring
   patterns of consonant harmony include:
   a. *Labial Assimilation (LA)* Assimilation of a nonlabial to a la-
      bial consonant; in most cases the consonant affected is al-
      veolar or palatal. Occurrences of labial assimilation seem to
      be evenly distributed between progressive and regressive
      patterns. Some examples are:

Progressive		**Regressive**	
pocket	papəp	zip	bɪp
boot	bup	jump	bʌmp

   b. *Velar Assimilation (VA)* Assimilation of a nonvelar to a velar
      consonant; in most cases the affected consonants are alveo-
      lar or palatal and the direction of assimilation is regressive:

Progressive		**Regressive**	
coat	kok	rock	gak
kiss	kɪk	jacket	gækət

   c. *Nasal Assimilation (NA)* Assimilation of a nonnasal to a na-
      sal consonant; place of articulation of the affected consonant
      may also be assimilated:

bunny	mʌni	done	nʌn
pink	mɪŋk	candy	næni

2. **Reduplication (Red)** Assimilation of one syllable to another,
   resulting in a reduplicated form:

water	wawa	noodle	nunu
bottle	baba	kitty	titi

3. **Voicing Assimilation** Appears in two forms:
   a. Voicing of an obstruent, usually a stop, in prevocalic posi-
      tion (PVc).
   b. Devoicing of an obstruent in final position, i.e., before a
      pause (FDvc).

Voicing		**Devoicing**	
pie	baɪ	bag	bæk
toe	do	bib	bɪp
kick	gɪk	nose	nos

   Even though they may devoice final consonants, some children maintain the voiced-voiceless distinction of the adult language by producing longer vowels in productions of words

ending in a voiced consonant. (As mentioned earlier, this same strategy has been observed in children who delete final consonants.) With vowel length as a distinctive feature, minimal pairs can be differentiated, e.g., *back* [bæk] versus *bag* [bæ:k], *duck* [dʌk] versus *dug* [dʌ:k].

Metathesis Before concluding this section, one additional error pattern needs to be mentioned: *metathesis.* Pronunciation errors attributed to metathesis involve the reordering, or transposition, of the consonantal elements of the target word. The following examples are cited in Smith (1973):

film	flɪm	elephant	ɛfələnt
alligator	ægəleitə	magnet	mæŋgɪt
animal	æmələn	mendable	mɛlbədən

Multiple Processes

Many examples of processes cited above are somewhat artificial in that they illustrate the occurrence of only a single process. In reality, target words are often affected by several processes at once, as shown in the examples below:

Word	Child's Form	Phonological Processes
drink	gɪk	CR (twice); VA
cheese	dit	PVc; S; FDvc
bottle	babu	LA; Voc
around	waʊn	USD; G; CR
small	ma	CR; FCD

In a few cases, phonological processes must be applied in a particular order if the child's pronunciation is to be described accurately. If the word *dog* is pronounced [gɔ], for example, the sound changes can be described as resulting from two processes, Velar Assimilation and Final Consonant Deletion. The processes must be applied in the order mentioned; if Final Consonant Deletion applied first, the resultant form would be [dɔ] (rather than [gɔ]) and Velar Assimilation could not apply. In the vast majority of cases, however, no ordering of processes is necessary.

Ages and Stages of Phonological Processes

Although the phonological processes described above have been well documented, little research has been directed toward determining the age, or age range, at which the various processes are present in the speech of normally developing children. The findings of various longitudinal studies involving single subjects or small groups of children and a few cross-sectional studies with larger subject populations (Crary et al., 1981; Hodson and Paden, 1981) provide a broad picture of the use of phonological processes at various chronological ages. Although there is considerable individual variation, phonological process occurrence can be divided into two major categories: processes that disappear by the age of 3;0 and those that persist beyond 3;0. Future research should permit us to break these categories down into more discrete age levels, but at this time the available data allow only the following division:

Processes Disappearing by 3;0	Processes Persisting after 3;0
Unstressed Syllable Deletion	Cluster Reduction
Final Consonant Deletion	Epenthesis
Doubling	Gliding
Diminutization	Vocalization
Velar Fronting	Stopping
Consonant Assimilation	Depalatalization
Reduplication	Final Devoicing
Prevocalic Voicing	

It should be noted that some of the processes in the left-hand column never occur in the speech of some children. In particular, Velar Fronting and the assimilation processes (e.g., Labial Assimilation, Velar Assimilation) evidence considerable variation, occurring frequently in the speech of some children but not at all in others (Vihman, 1978). The most widespread processes seem to be Unstressed Syllable Deletion, Final Consonant Deletion, Gliding, and Cluster Reduction, which are present in the speech of nearly all children.

Suppression, or disappearance, of a process may occur gradually, with application of the process being restricted to fewer and fewer target phonemes or to specific word positions. The process of *Cluster Reduction*, for example, might apply to all clusters in the early stages and then be restricted to final clusters, whereas *Stopping* might apply to all target fricatives at first, then only to a subset of fricatives. The phonemes /ð/ and /v/ are particularly prone to being produced as stops for an extended period, often until the child is 6;0 or older (Snow, 1963).

Although it is not yet possible to identify specific *ages* for the appearance and disappearance of various processes, sequential stages in the use of some processes have been observed. For example, final voiced stops are generally affected by two processes;

Table 2.6 Processes Affecting Initial Fricatives in Amahl Smith's Speech, Age 2;2–3;2[a]

Target Phoneme	Processes Used at Certain Ages						
	2;2	2;4	2;6	2;8	2;10	3;0	3;2
f-	GL	GL, FS	GL, C	GL, FS, C	ST, C	C	C
v-		GL, FS, C	GL, FS, C	GL, FS, C	GL, FS, C	GL, FS, C	GL, O, C
θ-	ST	GL, ST, O	ST	ST	ST, FS	FS	FS
ð-		ST	ST	ST	ST	ST	ST
s-	ST, DL	GL, ST, DL, O	GL, ST, DL, O	GL, ST, O, C	GL, ST, O, C	ST, C	C
z-	GL	GL, ST	GL, ST, O, C	GL, ST, O, C	ST, O, C	O, C	C
ʃ-	GL, ST, DL	GL, ST, DL	GL, ST	ST, Dep	ST, Dep, O, C	ST, Dep	Dep

Based on Smith (1973).

Key: GL = gliding; ST = stopping; DL = deletion; FS = fricative substitute; O = other process; Dep = depalatalization; C = correct.
[a]Substitutions involving only a change in voicing (e.g., s → z, f → v) are not included.

Final Consonant Deletion occurs first, then Final Consonant Devoicing. Clusters composed of /stop + liquid/ are potentially subject to three processes: (1) Cluster Reduction (e.g., /pl/ → [p]); (2) gliding (e.g., /pl/ → [pw]); and (3) Epenthesis (e.g., /pl/ → [pəl]). All children do not necessarily pass through each stage, but if the processes do occur they generally appear in the order mentioned.

Although it is tempting to posit discrete stages for the occurrence and disappearance of all the phonological processes, the longitudinal studies carried out to date do not provide evidence of such stages, particularly for the acquisition of fricative and affricate phonemes, and of clusters. Table 2.6 shows the processes affecting the initial fricatives produced by one child, Amahl Smith, between the ages of 2;2, when none of the target sounds were produced correctly, and 3;2 when several were pronounced correctly (Smith, 1973).

It can be seen that during the 12-month period there is no evidence of a smooth progression from one process to another; rather, a variety of processes co-occur during each 2-month interval shown. The most widespread processes, Stopping and Gliding, are present throughout the year, and for some sounds both occur during the same 2-month period. Edwards (1979) reported similar results in her longitudinal study of the acquisition of fricatives by six American children. Summarizing her findings, she stated: "There is no clear progression of substitution types in any given position, either for individual fricatives or for fricatives as a group; instead different types of substitutions co-occur."

The fluctuation and variation of phonological processes in the speech of Amahl Smith and reported in the results of other longitudinal studies highlight the problem of defining discrete stages of process use. It is our belief that at this time we do not have enough longitudinal data to make reliable statements regarding ages and stages of occurrence of processes in normally developing children. Future research, particularly longitudinal studies with larger numbers of subjects, will allow us to make more accurate statements regarding this topic.

Summary

It has been shown that between the ages of 1;6 and 8;0 normally developing children acquire the segmental and most of the suprasegmental elements of their language. In many cases segmental

development may be achieved by age 5;0 or 6;0, but suprasegmental development—particularly acquisition of adult-like timing—is typically not obtained until the age of 11;0 or 12;0 (Kent,
1976).

In spite of considerable individual variation, studies of segmental acquisition reveal general developmental patterns in terms
of place and manner of articulation of consonants. For *manner* of
articulation, the classes of nasals, stops, and glides are typically
acquired early, and fricatives, affricates, and liquids are learned
later. Analysis of incorrect productions show that the early-
acquired sound classes often serve as substitutes for classes acquired later; for instance, stops are substituted for fricatives and
affricates (the process of Stopping), and glides are substitutes for
liquids (the process of Gliding).

In terms of *place* of articulation, the most common pattern of
acquisition is front consonants before back ones: labial > alveolar > palatal and velar. Here again, consonants acquired early
often substitute for those learned later, e.g., alveolars for velars
(Velar Fronting) and alveolars for palatals (Depalatalization). There
is, however, a good deal of individual variation regarding places
of articulation. Some children acquire velar phones relatively early
(before age 2;0) and often substitute a velar for an alveolar consonant in certain phonetic contexts, e.g., *duck* is pronounced [gʌk]
(Velar Assimilation). Other children acquire velars relatively late
and tend to substitute alveolars for velars, e.g., *key* is pronounced
[ti] (Velar Fronting).

In terms of *syllabic shapes,* the CV syllable is typically acquired
first and is the most common syllabic type in the early stages of
acquisition, ages 1;0–1;6 (Winitz and Irwin, 1958). The closed syllable CVC appears somewhat later (ages 1;6–2;0), and in some
children's speech it occurs more frequently than the CV syllable
(Ingram, 1978). Two common error patterns contribute to the high
proportion of CV and CVC syllabic structures: Final Consonant
Deletion (e.g., *boat* pronounced [bo]) and Cluster Reduction (e.g.,
bread pronounced [bɛd]).

Chapter 3

The Process of Development

Careful descriptions of the segmental and suprasegmental features of child speech are an essential part of our understanding of phonological development. They provide us with valuable information regarding *what* children learn and *when* they learn it. However, even the most complete descriptions cannot give us a full understanding of the course of acquisition; they must be accompanied by research focusing on the underlying processes, research on *how* children learn their phonological system.

It is not always easy to separate *process* (how something is learned) from *product* (what is learned), and some of the topics introduced here have been touched on in Chapter 2. However, we believe that the topics presented in this chapter relate more to the *how* than the *what* of phonological development. The discussions here are admittedly somewhat "fuzzier" than those of Chapter 2 because we are dealing with *covert* rather than overt aspects of acquisition.

As a starting point for the discussion, consider the linguistic and phonological skills of a hypothetical 1-year-old, Sherry. In her home environment, Sherry is exposed to much speech, a portion of which is addressed directly to her. She understands about 40 words or simple phrases but produces only four or five words that have an identifiable adult model. In addition to her word productions, she babbles long strings of syllables with various intonational contours. In both babbling and meaningful speech, her productions are dominated by simple consonant–vowel (CV) syllables in which the consonant is usually a stop, nasal, or glide. At this stage, her productions are severely limited by a variety of factors, including motor control, perception, and cognitive/linguistic factors. By the age of 5, Sherry will have acquired a vocabulary of around 2,000 words and will be able to pronounce most sounds and sound sequences of English.

In order to accomplish this phenomenal task, she must have the ability to: (1) recognize and store new lexical items; (2) plan and execute the articulatory gestures needed for correct pronunciation of these items; and (3) compare the input (adult form) with her own output and then modify her pronunciation if the two forms do not match. Just how this is all achieved is not understood, but we do know something of the processes involved. The discussion that follows is divided into two major sections. The first focuses on phenomena related, in one way or another, to phonological acquisition; the second is devoted to a review and critique of theories of development.

Related Factors

Speech Motor Development

Although it is an important aspect of phonological development, relatively little is known about the acquisition of speech motor skills and even less about the role of these skills in the overall picture of development. Only now are researchers designing studies aimed at answering some of the basic questions involved. One thing is clear: speech motor acquisition differs from other aspects of development (e.g., linguistic, cognitive) in that it is a *skill* that undergoes a relatively long period of development, beginning at birth and ending around the onset of puberty. [For more complete discussions of this topic, the reader is referred to Kent (1980, 1981) and Netsell (1981).]

Motor development clearly plays a role in the mastery of correct production of speech sounds and sound sequences. Although there is as yet no real measure of articulatory difficulty, some sounds are intuitively "easier" to produce than others. Stops, nasals, glides, and vowels fall into the "easy-to-produce" category, whereas fricatives and affricates are more "difficult" to articulate. As shown in Chapter 2, "easy" sounds occur frequently in babbling and tend to be mastered early in meaningful speech, whereas "difficult" sounds appear rarely in babbling and are mastered much later. In terms of syllable shapes, the CV syllable is "easier" to articulate and is learned earlier than CVC syllables or syllables containing consonant clusters. In some sense, the articulatory gestures associated with "easy" sounds and syllable shapes are simpler and/or less precise than those required in the production of "more difficult" sound/syllable types.

Assimilatory patterns occurring in early productions can also be related to the notion of articulatory ease. As shown in Chapter 2, there are two major types of assimilation: consonantal assimilation (e.g., *duck* pronounced [gʌk]) and syllable assimilation (e.g., *water* pronounced [wawa].) It seems reasonable to assume that it is easier to produce a word composed of two identical syllables (e.g., [wawa]) or of one syllable with two similar consonants (e.g., [gʌk]) than a word with two or three different consonants. The occurrence of assimilatory patterns varies significantly across children, although it has been argued by some that reduplication (i.e., syllable assimilation) is universal (Fee and Ingram, 1982; Ferguson, 1978, 1983; Moskowitz, 1971).

Whereas mastery of articulatory gestures for most individual sounds is completed by the time children are age 5;0 or 6;0, full mastery of the dynamic, temporal aspects of speech production takes much longer. Kent (1981) noted that there are, in fact, two types of temporal learning that must take place. After the onset of meaningful speech, the child must learn to *sequence,* or temporally order, articulatory units as they are ordered in the adult model. For example, production of the word *soup* involves sequencing the articulatory gestures needed to articulate the phones [s], [u], and [p].

In addition to ordering the phones properly, the child must learn to *coarticulate* the articulatory movements to produce words with adult-like timing characteristics. In the word *soup,* for example, production of [s] is affected by the following [u], which in turn is affected by the final [p]. Spectrographic comparisons of adult and child productions indicate that anticipatory movements involved in coarticulation are much greater in adults than in children. Although sequencing seems to be mastered by the age of 3 or 4, coarticulation between sounds does not reach an adult-like state until 11 or 12 years (Kent, 1980).

The apparent lack of coarticulation in young children's speech has been interpreted as an inability to preprogram sequences of articulatory movements prior to their execution. Although preprogramming (also called motor programming) may not become fully adult-like until long after the onset of speech, there is evidence that such programming exists in the early stages of acquisition. As discussed in Chapter 2, one of the major types of phonological processes involves assimilations of one consonant to another. In monosyllabic words, the great majority of consonant assimilations are *regressive* (rather than progressive), meaning that a final consonant affects an initial consonant, e.g., *sock* [gak] (Velar Assimilation), *jump* [bʌmp] (Labial Assimilation), *spoon* [mun] (Nasal Assimilation). This pattern of assimilation indicates that children under the age of two do indeed employ some sort of motor programming in articulating words and phrases (see Stoel-Gammon, 1983a, for further examples). The programming may be very rudimentary, but it does seem to occur. Further research in this area is needed if we are to understand: (1) the development of coarticulation; and (2) the relationship between speech motor learning and phonological acquisition in general.

To provide a possible framework for such research, Netsell (1981) hypothesized three overlapping stages of speech motor development: (1) The first stage (birth to 2 years) centers around the control of *spatial* aspects—"the child is practicing placement, shaping, or movements of the components parts that yield acoustic patterns to approximate his model(s)." (2) The second stage (ages 1;0–6;0) focuses on *spatial–temporal* coordination—the child learns to combine the static, spatial aspects of articulation with the dynamic, temporal movements associated with the articulation of sounds and sound sequences. (3) The final stage, labeled the *temporal* period (ages 3;0–11;0), is dominated by the acquisition of adult-like timing—the child masters the anticipatory gestures underlying the coarticulation of sound sequences.

Phonological Strategies

During recent years a number of researchers have referred to "phonological strategies" children use when acquiring their phonological system (e.g., Farwell, 1977; Ferguson and Farwell, 1975; Kiparsky and Menn, 1977; Schwartz and Leonard, 1982; Vihman, 1981). Although there is no consensus on the exact definition of the term "strategy," it is generally agreed that phonological strategies allow children to organize and simplify the complex phonological system being acquired.

The notion of *lexical selection* (discussed in Chapter 2) is one example of a phonological strategy for dealing with early lexical and phonological acquisition. This strategy allows children to reduce the size and complexity of their early lexicon by limiting the phonological form of the adult words they try to produce. Thus a given child may attempt only words with initial stops or composed of reduplicated syllables. Another example of a phonological strategy is the widespread use of *homonymy* in early productions, e.g., Daniel's use of [gak] cited in Chapter 2. The presence of many homonymous forms has been interpreted as a strategy that allows the child to produce a large number of adult words using relatively few articulatory patterns (Stoel-Gammon and Cooper, 1981; Vihman, 1981). Thus in the case cited earlier, Daniel was able to include eight adult words in his productive vocabulary (*quack, rock, clock, sock, frog, yuk, block, milk*) and pronounce them all as [gak].

The use of *idiosyncratic rules* for dealing with multisyllabic words has also been described as a strategy. Priestly (1977) and Smith (1973) both noted that their sons developed unique ways of dealing with certain types of adult words. Between the ages of 1;10 and 2;2, Priestly's son created a single output pattern—[CVjVC]—for pronouncing some, but not all, polysyllabic words. As shown below, the initial and final consonants (C) of the pattern are clearly related to the consonantal elements of the adult form but not in an entirely systematic way, e.g.:

peanut	pijat	farmer	fajam
panda	pajan	seven	sɛjan
basket	bajak	lizard	zijan
turkey	tajak	rhinoceros	rajas

A different strategy for dealing with polysyllabic words was developed by Smith's son Amahl (age 3;4). He treated all words beginning with an unstressed syllable in a uniform manner by substituting the form [ri-] for the target syllable, e.g.:

attack	ritæk	thermometer	rimɔmitə
arrange	rireɪnz	adaptor	ridæptə
disturb	ristə:v	infection	rifɛksən
design	ridzaɪn	elastic	rilæstɪk

The use of rules such as these has been documented in only a few children and may occur infrequently. They should not be considered marginal to our discussion of strategies, however, but as another example of a basic tendency to simplify the phonological form of word productions. Viewed in this manner, idiosyncratic rules, as well as homonymy and lexical selection, can be interpreted as a means by which children reduce the complexity involved in the task of phonological acquisition.

In concluding, it should be pointed out that strategies represent one of the "fuzzier" aspects of phonological development.

Strategies are not easy to define and identify, making it difficult to determine their frequency of occurrence in child speech. In our view, strategies have both a cognitive/linguistic component and a speech motor component; children formulate strategies (cognitive/ linguistic component) in order to reduce the articulatory require- ments (speech motor component) associated with word produc- tion.

Phonetic Versus Phonological Acquisition

It was noted in Chapter 1 that acquisition of a phonological system entailed learning both the *phonetic* and *phonological* features of a language. Children must not only learn to articulate sounds and sound sequences correctly (phonetic mastery), they must also learn to use those sounds in accordance with the phonological patterns of the adult language (phonological learning). In many instances the two aspects of acquisition are not in synchrony, with pho- nological learning preceding phonetic mastery. To illustrate, take the case of /s/ and /ʃ/ and a child who is aware that they contrast phonemically but is unable to accurately produce that contrast phonetically. Some children simply produce the two phonemes as [s], thus losing the phonemic contrast. However, other children may produce the contrast using a dentalized [s̪] or a lateral fricative [ɬ] to represent the phoneme /ʃ/. In this way, the phonological opposition is maintained, although the phonetic form of the con- trast differs from that of the adult language.

Fey and Gandour (1982) described a child who developed a unique way of producing the voicing distinction between voiced and voiceless stops in final position. Unable to pronounce /b, d, g/ accurately in final position, their subject (age 1;9–2;2) produced them with a nasal release, thereby differentiating them from final /p, t, k/:

stub	dabm̩	big	bɪgŋ̍
feed	vidn̩	egg	ɛgŋ̍
bad	bædn̩		

There are also cases in which phonetic ability precedes phon- ological knowledge. Smith (1973) cited a child who consistently substituted [θ] for target /s/, saying [θɪk] for *sick*. At the same time, this child substituted [f] for /θ/, pronouncing *thick* as [fɪk]. The erroneous pronunciation of *thick* was not due to inability to pro- duce a phonetic target—the child could produce [θ], as shown by his rendition of *sick*—but to a mismatch between phonetic mastery and use of a phonetic target in accordance with the ambient language.

Advanced and Frozen Forms

Another example of a mismatch in the child's developing phonological system comes from the occurrence of *advanced forms,* sometimes called "phonological idioms" (Moskowitz, 1980), and *frozen forms.* Advanced forms are utterances that are pronounced more accurately than other utterances of the same period. To use an oft-cited example, Hildegard Leopold produced the word *pretty* as [prɪtʰi] at 0;11 (Leopold, 1947) at a time when none of her other utterances included initial clusters or aspirated stops. The occurrence of a form such as *pretty* provides support for the notion that in the first word stage the child's lexicon is word based rather than phoneme based (see discussion in Chapter 2).

Frozen forms are words whose pronunciation remains the same after changes in the child's phonological system make the pronunciation of phonetically similar words more adult-like. Consequently, these forms are more primitive than other productions of the same period. To illustrate, if a child continues to pronounce the word *blanket* as [kiki] after her other utterances are no longer affected by the processes of Reduplication and/or Velar Assimilation, her rendition of *blanket* would be considered a frozen form.

Gradual Nature of Acquisition

Both cross-sectional investigations of large groups of children (e.g., Olmsted, 1971) and longitudinal studies of small groups of children or single subjects (e.g., Edwards, 1978; Macken and Barton, 1980; Smith, 1973) have shown that speech sound acquisition is gradual rather than abrupt. Phonemes are mastered first in a few words, often in a particular word position, and then spread through the rest of the vocabulary. For example, Amahl Smith (Smith, 1973) first produced the phoneme /f/ correctly at around age 2;5 in only two or three words. In other lexical items, /f/ was most frequently produced as [w] in initial position and [p] or [ɸ] in final position. Three to four months later /f/ was produced correctly in the majority of words, although there was still some variation between [f], [w], and [ɸ] word initially, and [f] and [ɸ] word finally. At around age 2;10, nearly 5 months after its appearance, /f/ was a stable member of Amahl's phonetic inventory.

In some instances, considerable variation has been reported in young children's productions of a target phoneme, or target word, with accurate productions co-occurring with inaccurate ones. For example, Scollon (1976) recorded 10 successive repetitions of the word *shoe*—[ṣ], [ʃɪ], [ʃ], [ʃɪʃ], [su], [suʔ], [sus], [ʃi], [ʃɪ], [ʃuʔ]— produced by his subject at age 1;7. Even greater variation is present in Daniel's renditions of *orange*, produced over a 2-week period at about age 1;5: [ɔ̃i], [ũni], [nini], [ɔɪʃ], [otʰu], [õdʒ], [ɪni], [owənɪʃ], [owɪtʃ], [owɪʃ], [ori] (Stoel-Gammon and Cooper, 1981). Menn (1979) referred to the extreme variation in Daniel's production of *orange* as "floundering" and attributed it to the lack of a "well-formed rule for dealing with a particular string of phones."

A final aspect of the nature of acquisition comes from data revealing that development is not always characterized by a smooth progression toward adult-like pronunciations. As mentioned earlier, Hildegard (Leopold, 1947) pronounced *pretty* correctly at age 0;11; however, at 1;4 her pronunciation was less accurate, [pwɪti]; at 1;9 it was [pɪti]; and at 1;10 it was [bɪdi]. In essence, Hildegard's renditions of *pretty* had regressed from an *advanced form* to a pronunciation that conformed to the production patterns found in other utterances at age 1;10. Menn (1982) provided another example of a pronunciation that became less like the adult form. At one stage, her son pronounced *down* correctly as [dæwn] and *stone* as [don]; but later, after the introduction of a nasal harmony rule, both words were produced with an initial nasal: *down* [næwn] and *stone* [non]. Menn (1982) attributed the change in pronunciation to "overgeneralization" of a newly formed rule of nasal harmony. (See Macken and Ferguson, 1983, for a discussion of regression and overgeneralization in phonological development.)

Perception

Infant Speech Perception Phonological acquisition involves the perception as well as the production of the speech sounds of the ambient language. Studies of speech perception have shown that the perceptual capabilities of young babies are quite remarkable. By the age of 6 months, infants can discriminate many speech-sound contrasts ranging from distinctions in voice onset time (Eimas et al., 1971) and place of articulation (Eimas, 1974) to differences in syllable stress (Spring and Dale, 1975) and pitch contour (Morse, 1972). In addition, infants can recognize similarities among sounds even when these sounds occur in different phonetic contexts or when they are produced by different speakers (Kuhl, 1980).

Babies are not able to discriminate *all* speech-sound contrasts during the first year of life, however; in particular, contrasts within the class of fricatives have proved difficult. Eilers and Minifie (1975) reported that infants ages 1–4 months failed to distinguish [sa] from [za], and Eilers et al. (1977) found that 6- to 8-month-old infants could not discriminate between [fi] and [θi]. Kuhl (1979) suggested that failure to discriminate may be due to insufficient linguistic experience, the need for maturation, or a combination of the two.

In contrast to the findings of studies that show that babies' perceptual skills are well developed by the end of the first year, investigations of subjects ages 1;6–3;0 indicate that children in this age group have difficulty distinguishing speech-sound contrasts that were easily discriminated at a younger age. These discrepant findings, although apparently contradictory, can be attributed to the fact that *linguistic* perception is much more complex than *speech-sound discrimination* tested in infants.

In most infant studies, subjects are presented with stimulus pairs that differ in only one phonetic feature—e.g., [sa] versus [za], [la] versus [ra], ['baba] versus [ba'ba]—and evidence of discrimination is based on a behavioral change in the infant (e.g., an increase in the rate of sucking or a turn of the head) when a new stimulus is presented. Thus the studies assess the ability to detect differences between acoustically similar stimuli. With older children, the experimental procedure is quite different. Subjects are presented with objects (or pictures) that are paired with phonetically similar labels. In some studies the labels are nonsense forms, e.g., [fɪs] versus [θɪs]; in others they are real words, e.g., *bear* versus *pear* (see discussion below). The children are then required to demonstrate that they know which label is associated with which object. To succeed in this task, the child must not only be able to discriminate between acoustically similar stimuli, but also to use the sound contrasts *linguistically* by associating them with objects in the real world. Whereas speech-sound discrimination is present in infancy, linguistic use of sound contrasts involves the classification of sounds into phonemes and requires more memory and considerably more exposure to the mother tongue.

Linguistic Perception The first experimental study of phonemic perception was carried out in 1949 by Shvachkin (English translation, 1973), a Russian psychologist who developed a unique procedure for testing young children. He taught each child nonsense CVC labels for three objects, e.g., *mak, bak, zub;* in each set, two of the labels were minimal pairs (i.e., differed in only one segment). The labels were taught one at a time, and once they were learned the child was presented with all three objects and asked to perform an action, e.g., "Give me *mak*"; "Point to the *bak*." The study was longitudinal and involved 18 subjects ages 0;10–1;6 at the beginning of data collection and 1;6–2;0 at the end.

Shvachkin (1973) reported that his subjects were *not* capable of perceiving all the phonemic contrasts at the earliest age and that the development of phonemic perception proceeded in a regular fashion across his subject population. On the basis of his findings, he posited a universal order of acquisition of perception of speech-sound contrasts:

Level 1: distinction among vowels
Level 2: presence versus absence of consonants
Level 3: sonorants (liquids, nasals, glides) versus voiced stops
Level 4: palatalized versus nonpalatalized consonants
Level 5: distinction among sonorants
Level 6: distinction among obstruents (stops, fricatives)

Nearly 25 years after the Russian study, Garnica (1973) used Shvachkin's testing techniques to study phonemic perception in English-speaking children. Although her subjects displayed greater variability than the Russian children and were not able to perceive certain phonemic contrasts by 2 years of age, her findings provide support for the general stages of acquisition posited by Shvachkin.

On the basis of these studies, it seems that: (1) phonemic perception is not fully developed at the onset of meaningful speech (around 12–15 months); and (2) there is a regular order of acquisition for the phonemic perception of speech-sound contrasts. However, further research has cast doubt on these conclusions. First, Barton (1975) reanalyzed Garnica's data using a more conservative statistical treatment and showed that there was little or no support for hypothesizing a universal order of acquisition. He then designed his own study of phonemic perception in English-speaking children (Barton, 1976) testing subjects between ages 2;3 and 2;11. His findings reveal that *word familiarity* plays an important role in phonemic perception. When his subjects already knew the word labels for the objects they were asked to discriminate, they were able to perceive sound contrasts that had proved difficult for the children in Garnica's study.

In a second study, Barton (1976) showed that younger children, ages 1;8–2;0, were able to discriminate the voicing contrast between two pairs of familiar words: *pear–bear* and *coat–goat*. This contrast was tested because Garnica (1973) had reported that it was acquired relatively late in her subjects.

The effect of word familiarity on phonemic perception was further examined by Clumeck (1982), who used a picture-pointing task to assess discrimination of minimal word pairs. He tested 30 children, ages 3;1–5;10, and found that the younger children were unable to identify phonemic distinctions when the stimulus pairs contained unfamiliar words; for example, they could distinguish between /p/ and /k/ in the word-pair *peas–keys* but not in the pair *pouch–couch*. Overall, the 3-year-old subjects failed to recognize a contrast in 90% of the instances when an unfamiliar word was used, compared with a failure rate of 3.5% for familiar words. Among the older subjects, the effect of word familiarity was evident but was much diminished. The 5-year-olds were unable to discriminate 30% of the pairs containing unfamiliar words; when familiar words were tested, the failure rate was less than 1%.

Although this study provides convincing evidence that phonemic perception is greatly influenced by a child's receptive vocabulary, this does not necesssarily mean that perception is fully developed at the onset of meaningful speech as Barton (1976), Smith (1973), and others have claimed. As Clumeck (1982) pointed out in the conclusion of his study, his findings of age-related differences in phonemic perception indicate that "children's phoneme identification abilities may not become adult-like until several years after they have begun speaking." In light of the divergent results from studies of perception in children ages 3;0–8;0 (see Barton, 1980, for a review), more research is needed before truly definitive statements can be made regarding the development of perception after the onset of speech.

Perception and Production As might be expected given the preceding discussion, the relationship between children's perception of phonological contrasts and their production of those contrasts is not well understood. Several hypotheses regarding this relationship have been proposed, ranging from Straight's (1980) claim that perception and production are distinct and independent components of the language acquisition process to Smith's contention (1973) that perception precedes production, to Shvachkin's belief (1973) that correct production can precede and facilitate perception of certain sounds.

The major issue in understanding the relationship between perception and production is this: Do children perceive speech in terms of adult phonological distinctions, in terms of their own systems, or somewhere in between? Advocates in favor of the first hypothesis claim that children are capable of perceiving speech-sound contrasts in an adult-like manner well before they are able to produce them; the task during the period of acquisition, then, is to learn to produce those contrasts. Smith (1973) is a proponent of this theoretical position, basing his arguments on data from his son Amahl. He first noted that prior to the onset of speech Amahl was able to distinguish minimal word pairs. Later, through informal testing with picture cards, Smith was able to ascertain that the boy could discriminate between word pairs such as *mouse–mouth* and *card–cart* even though they were produced as homophones. On the basis of his observations, Smith concluded that: "I would hypothesize that the child doesn't begin to speak until he has learnt to perceive at least the majority of the contrasts present in the adult language." Although the data from Amahl show that perception may well precede production (at least for some sound contrasts), they are not sufficient to warrant the claim that phonemic perception is complete, or nearly complete, prior to the onset of speech.

According to the alternative hypotheses, perceptual skills are still developing during the period of meaningful speech, and production errors may be direct reflections of perceptual confusion. Thus if a child fails to produce the /w-r/ contrast in *wing* and *ring*, pronouncing them both [wɪŋ], it may be that he is unable to perceive the distinction between /w/ and /r/ in adult speech. Several experimental studies (e.g., Locke, 1980b; Menyuk, 1980) provide data to support this hypothesis by showing that in some cases failure to produce a phonemic contrast is associated with the inability to perceive that contrast. Perceptual confusions as the basis for production errors seem to be more frequent among fricative phonemes, particularly /f/ versus /θ/, than among other sound classes (Edwards, 1974; Eilers and Oller, 1976; Johnson and Hardee, 1981).

Given the evidence currently available, it seems that in some, perhaps most, cases it can be shown that perception of speech-sound contrasts precedes their production. In a few cases, however, production errors can be directly related to perceptual confusion.

Underlying Representations

A final issue related to perception and production is the way in which children internally store words that are part of their vocabulary, usually referred to as the child's underlying (or internal) lexical representation. This aspect of a child's linguistic system is exceedingly difficult to study because it cannot be tested directly but must be inferred from observations of perceptual and productive abilities. It has been argued that there are two possibilities for the child's underlying representation: it is based on either the *adult spoken form* or the *child's own pronunciation*.

Smith (1973) stated unequivocally that the first alternative is correct, basing his claim primarily on the "across-the-board" nature of phonological change: "when a child learns to pronounce a new sound or combination of sounds he immediately utilizes it correctly in all relevant words, rather than adding it piecemeal to each word as he re-hears it." Because of the rapidity involved in the change, Smith inferred that "the sounds and sound sequences [of the adult words] must have been stored in the brain 'correctly' in order for their appearance to be so consistently right." According to this hypothesis, a child who regularly substituted [p] for initial /f/ would modify his pronunciation of all *f*-initial words once he learned to articulate the fricative correctly.

Both Braine (1976) and Macken (1980b) examined Smith's analyses in some detail and questioned his statements regarding the "across-the-board" nature of *all* phonological changes. They concluded that, although many lexical items are stored in the adult surface (i.e., spoken) form, there are cases in which the child misperceives a word or set of words and consequently stores it incorrectly.

Another aspect of Smith's hypotheses that needs to be questioned is his unstated assumption that the perceived form and the underlying representation are the same. Although this may indeed be the case, it should not be taken for granted. As shown below, there is the potential for a variety of relationships between the perceived and the stored form:

1. It may be, as Smith (1973) suggested, that the child perceives an adult word correctly and stores it in the adult spoken form.
2. The child may perceive the adult word correctly but store it in a *simplified* form with features or segments altered or omitted (Ingram, 1976; Waterson, 1971).
3. The child may perceive a word incorrectly and store it in its misperceived form (Macken, 1980b).
4. The child may have two underlying representations, one for comprehension based on perception of the adult word and one for production based on his own pronunciation (Straight, 1980).

This is not intended to be an exhaustive list of possible relationships but to show that we should not simply assume that the perceived form and underlying representations are the same.

Dinnsen and his colleagues (Dinnsen, 1984; Dinnsen et al., 1979; Maxwell, 1982) attempted to formulate some general procedures for determining if a child's underlying representation matched the adult spoken form. For example, to decide if a child who regularly omits final consonants has any (productive) "knowledge" of the consonant in question, Dinnsen suggested that the child's productions be analyzed in terms of morphophonemic alternations and/or free variation that would indicate knowledge of the consonant; in addition, acoustic measurements of segment durations could be performed. If the analyses show that the child who produces *dog* as [da], pronounces *doggie* as [dagi] (rather than [daịi]), or produces *dog* variably as [da] or [dag], it is concluded that his underlying form includes a final /g/. If, on the other hand, there are no instances of free variation, no morphophonemic alternations, and no acoustic measurements indicating distinct forms in the child's pronunciation, it is assumed that he has no knowledge of the final consonant of the adult word and that his underlying representation closely resembles his own spoken form.

Although these guidelines appeared to work well for the group of language-disordered subjects studied by Dinnsen et al., some caution must be taken in using them with younger, normally developing children, because the "knowledge" of an older child (age 3;6–5;0) with a disordered phonological system should not be directly equated with that of a young normal child just learning to talk. Further research is needed in this area to determine the validity of the approach. In addition, our understanding of underlying representations should be linked not only to aspects of production, as it is in Dinnsen's work, but also to perception. Figure 3.1 presents a diagram of the way in which the relationship between perception, underlying representation, and production might be viewed. The figure is divided into two levels, differentiating the *overt* (observable) phenomena from the *covert* (unobservable) phonemena. Whenever the *output* (i.e., child's pronunciation) differs from the *input* (adult model), we should try to determine which stage or stages of the covert level were responsible for the lack of a match between the two forms.

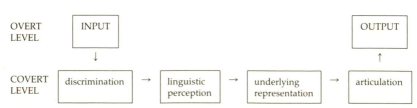

Figure 3.1 Relationship of perception and production.

Input

Although a number of studies have addressed the question of the relationship between input and syntactic, semantic, and/or pragmatic development (Snow and Ferguson, 1977), little research has been directed toward relating input to phonological acquisition. Obviously, input is important: if a child does not hear speech, he will not learn to talk; if he hears Chinese, he will speak Chinese. Beyond this, little is known.

There are two basic issues that need to be investigated: (1) What is the phonological nature of speech addressed to children? and (2) What is the relationship between input and phonological development? We know something about the first question but almost nothing about the second. A number of studies have shown that adults make phonological modifications when speaking to children. Ferguson (1964) noted that, in English, "baby talk" words are often reduplicated, e.g., *bye-bye, pee-pee, night-night,* or are phonetically simple forms, e.g., *tummy* (for *stomach*), *bunny* (for *rabbit*). In addition to simplifying their vocabulary, adults also tend to speak more slowly and articulate more clearly when addressing children (Bernstein-Ratner, 1983; Malsheen, 1980; Stoel-Gammon, 1983b). In particular, stressed items are often pronounced with great precision, e.g., *water* [watʰɚ] (rather than [waɾɚ]), *big* [bɪgə] (rather than [bɪg]).

Although descriptions of adult speech to children show that, at least in some instances, it is phonetically simpler and more carefully articulated than adult–adult speech, the effect of the simplifications on phonological acquisition is simply not known. They may help the child: (1) segment an utterance into words; (2) form an underlying representation; (3) produce a word more accurately; or (4) all, some, or none of these. Only future research will provide the answers.

Conclusion

In contrast to Chapter 2, which focused on the similarities observed in patterns of acquisition, this discussion of factors involved in the process of acquisition has highlighted *differences* in development. Given the possibility of differences in the use of phonological strategies, the occurrence of advanced and frozen forms, the types of mismatches between phonetic and phonological learning, and the construction of underlying forms, among others, it is not surprising that no two children acquire their phonological systems in precisely the same manner. In order to fully understand phonological development, both the similarities and the differences must be accounted for. As shown in the following section, none of the current theories meet this basic goal.

Theories of Phonological Development

Several theories have been proposed to account for the process of phonological development; they differ in fundamental ways, and thus far none has proved entirely satisfactory. The following section provides a brief description of the current theories, presented in chronological order. For a more detailed discussion of some of these theories, the reader is referred to Ferguson and Garnica (1975) and Menn (1982).

Requirements of a Theory

Before discussing the current theories of phonological development, it is useful to consider what we should expect of an adequate theory. Just what should a theory of phonological development do? In our opinion, it should fulfill the following requirements:

1. It should account for the body of factual information we have gathered about phonological acquisition. To meet this requirement, the theory must account for the *general patterns* that occur as well as the *individual differences* observed in order of acquisition, the use of phonological strategies, the occurrence of phonological processes, the presence of advanced forms, etc. It must also account for changes over time, both those that result in loss of a phonemic contrast and/or a decrease in phonetic accuracy and those that establish new phonemic contrasts and/or increase phonetic accuracy. Finally, it must explain the role of input and account for the relationship between prelinguistic (i.e., babbling) and linguistic development.
2. It must account for phonetic as well as phonological learning and must be able to explain the mismatches that often occur between the two.
3. It must be consistent with theories of speech perception and must account for the relationship between perception and production in phonological acquisition.
4. It must be compatible with other theories of learning, partic-

ularly theories of cognitive and general linguistic development.

5. It must be compatible with phonological theory.
6. It must make testable predictions regarding patterns of acquisition and error types.

Current Theories

Structuralist Theory The structuralist theory, proposed by Jakobson in 1941 (English translation, 1968), postulated a relationship between phonological acquisition in children, phonological universals of the languages of the world, and phonological dissolution with aphasia. According to the theory, there are two distinct periods of vocal productions: babbling and meaningful speech. During the babbling period, the child's productions are "ephemeral" and include "an astonishing quantity and diversity of sound productions" that do not follow any regular sequence of acquisition. With the onset of meaningful speech, the second period, the sound repertoire is severely reduced and speech sounds must be reacquired as part of the phonemic system of the child's native tongue.

During the second period, phonological development follows a universal and innate order of acquisition regulated by a hierarchical set of structural laws. The child begins with two very different sounds, a "wide" vowel /a/ and a "front articulated stop . . . generally a labial." Thereafter acquisition proceeds in an orderly fashion from "simple and undifferentiated to stratified and differentiated." Although the rate of acquisition may vary from child to child, the relative order of phonemic acquisition is said to be invariant.

According to Jakobson, acquisition entails the learning of feature contrasts rather than of sounds. The first contrast acquired is *consonantal–vocalic* (/p/–/a/); this is followed by the consonantal contrast *nasal–oral* (/p/–/m/) and then by *grave–acute* (labial–alveolar) (/p/–/t/). These two consonantal contrasts provide the child with a repertoire of four consonants (/p, t, m, n/) in the early stages of acquisition. For all children, the contrasts that differentiate stops and nasals are said to be acquired before those that differentiate fricatives, affricates, and liquids.

To some extent, Jakobson's theory has received support from longitudinal case studies (e.g., Leopold, 1947; Pačesova, 1968; Velten, 1943) and large-group cross-sectional studies (e.g., Templin, 1957). As predicted by the structuralist theory, most children acquire the classes of stops and nasals before fricatives, affricates, and liquids, and front consonants before back ones. These patterns, however frequent, are *not* universal. They are, at best, probabilistic rather than absolute.

Although studies of order of acquisition provide support for some aspects of Jakobson's theory, there is strong evidence to refute other aspects. First, investigations of the relationship between babbling and meaningful speech (Oller et al., 1976; Stoel-Gammon and Cooper, 1981; Vihman et al., 1981) reveal that they are not two distinct and independent periods of development but, rather, that they share common properties of phonetic repertoire and syllable shapes. Second, the presence of extensive individual variation in the order of phonemic acquisition and use of phonological strategies, etc. does not support the claim that all children adhere to an "innate" and "universal" course of acquisition. Finally, Jakobson seemed to assume that development proceeds in terms of phonemes and phonemic contrasts from the earliest stages of meaningful speech; however, studies of early word production indicate that, initially, contrasts may be between whole words or perhaps syllables rather than phonemes (Ferguson and Farwell, 1975).

Behaviorist Theory The behaviorist theory, introduced by Mowrer (1952, 1960) and adapted by Winitz (1969) and Olmsted (1966, 1971), emphasizes the role of contingent reinforcement in phonological acquisition and is general enough to account for the speech of "talking birds" as well as children. According to Mowrer (1952), the following steps are involved:

1. The infant identifies with the caretaker (usually the mother) and attends to her vocalizations during periods of feeding and general nurturing.
2. The infant associates the mother's speech with the primary reinforcements of food and care; as a result, her speech acquires secondary reinforcing properties.
3. The infant's speech-like vocalizations, being similar to the mother's, take on secondary reinforcing values of their own.
4. The infant's productions that most closely resemble adult speech are selectively reinforced by the mother and the infant.

Proceeding through these steps, infant vocalizations are shaped so that they conform more and more to the speech patterns of the adults in the immediate environment.

Mowrer's theory fulfills some of the requirements listed earlier, i.e., being compatible with other theories of learning (behavior-modification theory) and relating phonological development of the period of meaningful speech to that of babbling. The theory has a major flaw, however, in that it fails to meet the first requirement: it does not account for the data on hand. First, there is virtually no evidence to support the claim that reinforcement is the primary force in speech-sound acquisition. Deaf infants, unable to hear their own vocalizations or those of their parents, nevertheless babble much like hearing infants during the first year of life in spite of a lack of reinforcement. Second, there is no evidence that mothers selectively reinforce those vocalizations which resemble adult speech. Finally, according to this theory, phonological acquisition involves external shaping of vocal responses in the same way that an animal's responses are shaped through behavior modification. This view—that acquisition is an automatic and mechanistic form of learning—is not compatible with studies (previously cited) indicating that children take an active and creative role in learning their sound system.

Ease of Perception Theory Although Olmsted (1966, 1971) agreed with Mowrer's notion that contingent reinforcement played a crucial role in phonological acquisition, he argued that two additional factors must be taken into consideration: frequency of the various phonemes in the adult spoken language and ease of perceptibility of the phonemes. In a tightly woven argument based on definitions, postulates, theorems, and corollaries, Olmsted (1966) claimed, first, that those phones which occur most frequently in "ordinary" adult speech also occur most frequently in speech directed to children. Because these phones acquire reinforcing properties, the more frequently they occur in the input the more likely they are to appear in the child's productions. Second, it was claimed that "some phones are more discriminable than others" and that phones whose articulatory "components" (e.g., voicing, friction, nasality) are more discriminable are likely to be learned (i.e., produced correctly) earlier than phones whose components are less discriminable.

Using data from a study of perceptual confusion in adults (Miller and Nicely, 1955), Olmsted postulated that in English the components of voicing and nasality are more easily discriminable than friction and duration, which in turn are more discriminable than place of articulation. On the basis of this hierarchy, he then predicted that during the course of acquisition children would make more errors regarding place of articulation than friction or duration, more errors in place of articulation, friction, and duration than in voicing or nasality, and approximately the same number in voicing and nasality.

Olmsted's theory is commendable in that: (1) it recognizes the importance of input and perception for an adequate model of phonological development; and (2) it makes testable predictions. In many cases, however, his predictions regarding order of acquisition and frequency of error types have not been supported by empirical studies. Even his own investigation of the development of 100 children failed to support the theory (Olmsted, 1971). In particular, the postulated hierarchy of errors (place of articulation > friction and duration > voicing and nasality) was not borne out. Olmsted (1971) noted that his basic assumption that "predictions of error and success would be simple opposites of each other" is unfounded and must be abandoned.

Natural Phonology Theory Central to the theory of natural phonology (Stampe, 1969, 1973) is the notion of phonological process, defined by Stampe (1969) as a mental operation that "merges a potential phonological opposition into that member of the opposition which least tries the restrictions of the human speech capacity." The processes, described as being innate and universal, are said to be "natural" because they represent "natural responses to phonetic forces implicit in the human capacity for speech" (Donegan and Stampe, 1979). According to the theory, children do not actually acquire or develop a phonological system; rather, they learn to suppress or constrain those processes that do not occur in their language. For example, children acquiring English must learn to suppress the process of Final Devoicing, because English has both voiced and voiceless obstruents in word-final position, e.g. *back–bag, hiss–his*. In contrast, Vietnamese-learning children never need to suppress the devoicing process, because all final obstruents are voiceless in their language.

During the course of phonological acquisition, children constrain processes by *suppressing, limiting,* or *reordering* them. An example of each of these is given below; the form(s) shown in stage 1 represent productions before the process is constrained, and the forms for stage 2 show the changes that have occurred.

1. Suppression of the process of *Cluster Reduction:*

Target	Form	Stage 1	Stage 2
blue	[blu]	bu	blu
bread	[brɛd]	bɛd	brɛd

2. Limitation of the process of *Final Devoicing* so that it applies only to stops:

Target	Form	Stage 1	Stage 2
nose	[noz]	nos	noz
give	[gɪv]	gɪf	gɪv
mud	[mʌd]	mʌt	mʌt
bag	[bæg]	bæk	bæk

3. Reordering the process of *Velar Assimilation* (VA) and *Final Consonant Deletion* (FCD) so that the former applies after the latter:

Target	Form	Stage 1	Stage 2
dog	[dɔg]	VA gɔg	FCD dɔ
		FCD gɔ	VA not applicable

Stampe's theory has been adopted by many researchers in the field of child phonology, particularly the notion of phonological processes as a means of describing systematic errors occurring in the child's productions. In spite of the obvious enthusiasm for this approach, there are some important issues that remain unresolved. First there is Stampe's definition of phonological process. Although phonological processes provide a good method for describing error patterns, there is as yet no firm evidence that they are in fact "mental operations" as Stampe claimed. The problem with this issue (and with the claim itself) is that it is difficult to determine what kind of evidence would support (or refute) the notion of a process as a "mental operation."

A second concern is Stampe's belief that the child's underlying representation of a word is the same as the adult spoken form. If this were true, the child's perceptual system would have to be fully developed at the onset of meaningful speech. At this point, we do not know enough about children's underlying representations or their perceptual systems to make definitive statements regarding their status (see discussion, this chapter).

Finally, according to Stampe's theory, the child plays a relatively passive role in the process of phonological acquisition, with verbal productions governed by a system of innate, universal phonological processes. Children do not actively learn a particular phonological system; rather, they learn to suppress the application of those processes that do not occur in the adult language. The resultant system represents a "residue" of the set of innate processes found in the infant. This view is not compatible with findings of studies that show that the child is an active participant in phonological acquisition as evidenced by lexical selection, phonological strategies, etc.

Prosodic Theory The prosodic theory, proposed by Waterson (1970, 1971) assumes that speech perception, as well as production, is still developing during the early stages of language acquisition. According to the theory, children tend to perceive utterances as unanalyzed units, rather than as sequences of segments; upon hearing an utterance, they attend to and subsequently attempt to reproduce the most "salient" features of the utterance. Using a feature set that includes both segmental and suprasegmental features, Waterson (1971) described utterances in terms of their syllabic structure, stress pattern, and segmental characteristics, e.g., continuance, nasality, and sibilance. The words *finger, another, window,* and *Randall,* for example, are said to share the features of continuance, nasality, nonrounded syllable, voiced ending of all syllables, voiced onset of the second syllable, and prominence of the penultimate syllable.

Waterson postulated that children perceive the similarities in the structural and segmental patterns of groups of words such as those cited above and reproduce them with an output pattern that duplicates the salient features rather than the specific sound sequences. For example, her son produced the words *finger, another, window,* and *Randall* with a single basic form [ˈɲVɲV] (V = vowel), maintaining the nasality, syllabic structure, and stress pattern of the adult forms.

The prosodic theory has several strengths. First, it provides a means for explaining the lack of systematic correspondences between a target phoneme and its pronunciation by the child. If adult forms are perceived in terms of broad features rather than phonemic units, it is not unexpected that a phoneme will be treated differently in different lexical forms. Second, unlike the theories previously examined, it can account for extensive individual differences in the early stages of acquisition. Third, it considers perception and adult input as important factors of phonological development.

The theory is not entirely satisfactory, however, primarily because of its limited scope. It is based on a small corpus from one young child and deals only with the initial stages of acquisition. It does not account for general patterns of acquisition that have been reported, nor does it make predictions regarding order of acquisition or error types.

Cognitive Theory The cognitive theory, developed by Ferguson and his students, was described most completely by Macken and Ferguson (1983; see also Ferguson, 1978). The authors believed that the "universalist-linguistic" framework adopted by Jakobson (1968) and Stampe (1969, 1973), among others, fails to accommodate two important aspects of phonological acquisition: (1) the presence of widespread individual differences among children acquiring the same language; and (2) longitudinal research that shows that acquisition is not "a linear progression of unfolding abilities."

In order to account for these phenomena, Macken and Ferguson proposed a *cognitive* model of acquisition based on the premise that children play an *active* role in the acquisition process by formulating and testing hypotheses regarding the sound system being acquired. In support of the model, the authors cited the following behaviors:

1. In the early stages of meaningful speech production, children *selectively* attend to the language addressed to them and choose words with certain phonological characteristics for inclusion in their lexicon while avoiding words with other characteristics.
2. Children are *creative* in acquiring their phonology, as evidenced by the production of phonetic segments and word-like forms not found in the adult language.
3. Children *formulate hypotheses* about the phonological system being acquired and then *test* and *revise* these hypotheses on the basis of linguistic experience.

As evidence of hypothesis formation and hypothesis testing, the authors cited examples of overgeneralization, regression, and experimentation that have been observed in individual children.

The cognitive model focuses primarily on the early stages of phonological development when individual differences are greatest. It postulates that during the initial phases of acquisition children treat words as unanalyzed wholes rather than as sequences of segments. As their receptive and productive vocabulary increases, they begin to notice similarities between segments that belong to a particular sound class or between sequences of segments, and they formulate rules for relating words with similar sounds and/or syllabic shapes. The rules may vary from child to child, and even within a single child there is not always a steady progression toward the adult form because conflicting rules and competing hypotheses may cause a form to diverge more from the adult model than during the previous stage. Although they focused on individual differences, Macken and Ferguson did acknowledge that there are some universal or near-universal patterns in children's speech. They attributed these commonly occurring patterns to the universal nature of the auditory and articulatory systems of children and did not believe that their presence conflicts with the cognitive model of acquisition they have developed.

Menn (1976a; see also Kiparsky and Menn, 1977) proposed the "interactionist-discovery" theory of phonological development, which shares many features with the cognitive theory described here. Phonological acquisition is viewed as a "problem-solving" activity in which the child plays a central role. Although the two theories are highly similar, with both stressing the child's creativity, Menn paid more attention to the dichotomy between phonetic and phonological learning, hypothesizing that in the early stages words are learned as unanalyzable *phonetic* forms. Subsequently, these words are segmented and reorganized on the basis of phonemes.

Like Waterson's prosodic theory (1971), the cognitive theory can easily account for individual differences in early development. It goes further than the prosodic theory in providing explanations for phenomena not considered in most other theories, e.g., lexical selection, regression, the use of phonological strategies, etc. Although its coverage of the early stages of development is outstanding, it pays little attention to other, equally important issues, e.g., (1) later development; (2) the relationship of perception and production; and (3) the similarities (general patterns) observed in studies of large groups of subjects. In addition, it fails to make testable predictions regarding phonological development.

Biological Theory Locke (1980c; 1983b) proposed a model of phonological acquisition that emphasizes the similarities between the phonological patterns of late babbling and those of early meaningful speech. The model has three basic premises:

1. The prelinguistic vocalizations of infants from all linguistic environments are highly similar; during the late babbling period, more than 90% of the consonant-like phones produced are stops, nasals, and glides, whereas fricatives, affricates, and liquids account for fewer than 10% of the productions.
2. The phonetic repertoire and phonological patterns of early meaningful speech resemble closely those of the late babbling period; because the babbling patterns are universal, so are the patterns of the first words.
3. When substitutions occur in the child's productions, frequently occurring sounds from the babbling repertoire (i.e., stops, nasals, glides) serve as substitutes for infrequent babbling sounds (i.e., fricatives, affricates, liquids). The exact substitution patterns depend on perceptual similarity between frequent and infrequent segments. Locke used data on adult perceptual confusions (Wang and Bilger, 1973) to predict, for example, that [b] would substitute for /v/ and [d] for /ð/.

According to the model (Locke, 1983b), there are three major stages of phonological acquisition. During the *prelinguistic stage* infants come to realize that their vocalizations are capable of conveying information regarding basic needs or desires; their productions can be recognized as requests, calls, etc. Proto-words (i.e., word-like forms not based on an adult model) may appear toward the end of this stage.

The *second stage* begins when the child attempts to produce conventional words. Phonetically, these productions are much like those of the previous stage; phonologically they are different. Meaningful speech, unlike babbling, involves cognitive processes such as recognition of adult forms, storage and retrieval of words, and pattern matching, which were not needed in babbling. The *third stage* is characterized by marked changes in the child's phonological system. The sounds and sound patterns of meaningful speech no longer resemble those of babbling and become increasingly similar to those of the adult phonological system being acquired. During this stage vocabulary increases rapidly and the child begins to produce words with increasing phonological complexity. As the system develops, phonological acquisition ceases to be dominated solely by phonetic (or biological) tendencies. Instead, an interaction of *phonetic* and *cognitive* factors allows the possibility of individual differences in the course of development.

The strengths of Locke's theory are that it: (1) relates the phonological development of the prelinguistic and linguistic periods; (2) provides a partial explanation of the relationship between perception and production; (3) accounts for the similar developmental processes observed across children from different linguistic environments; and (4) attempts to relate the phonetic and cognitive components of acquisition.

Weaknesses of this theory can be attributed, in part, to the emphasis given to universal or near-universal patterns of development. Little attention is given to studies showing early individual differences in acquisition (e.g., Stoel-Gammon and Cooper, 1981, 1984; Vihman et al., 1981), and the use of phonological strategies in the early stages is not discussed. Here again, as in some of the previously cited theories, it seems to be assumed that in the early stages the child plays a passive rather than an active role in the process of phonological development.

Discussion

Although each theory meets some of the requirements outlined at the beginning of this section, none fulfills all of them. In particular, no theory adequately fulfills the first requirement—that a theory must account for both general patterns (i.e., similarities) and individual differences. Several theories, e.g., those of Jakobson, Stampe, and Olmsted (also Locke to some extent), focus almost exclusively on the similarities that occur. Although differing in detail, they all view development as an unfolding of innate capabilities. In contrast, the theories proposed by Waterson, Macken and Ferguson, and Menn pay little attention to similarities, stressing instead individual differences and the active, creative role children play in learning their phonological system.

The proposals of the two groups are not as incompatible as they might appear—they are merely focusing on different aspects of the same issue. It is undeniable that there are some universal or near-universal patterns, both in the order of acquisition of sound classes and syllable structures and in the types of errors that occur. At the same time, there is clear evidence that children do not follow a single path in learning to pronounce. The differences that have been documented can best be explained by a more cognitive approach. One way of reconciling the two theoretical positions is by positing a common core based on features of articulatory and perceptual systems and on maturational growth. This common core, which is responsible for general patterns, functions in conjunction with the child's cognitive system, allowing him to recognize, store, and produce utterances, and to form and test hypotheses regarding the phonological system being acquired.

Because the common core interacts with the cognitive system, children's "solutions" to the problem of producing a sound or sound sequence are often the same. For example, take the case of consonant clusters. Given that it is easier to produce a single consonant than a sequence of consonants (because of characteristics of the articulatory system), children tend to simplify consonant clusters. Many children simply omit one of the consonants, usually the one that is more difficult to pronounce; thus *snow* is pronounced [no] and *blow* is [bo] in accordance with the most common pattern. However, some children simplify clusters in other ways; they may, for example, insert a vowel between the two consonants, thereby breaking up the cluster, e.g., *blow* [bəlo], they may move one consonant to another part of the word, e.g., *snow* [nos], or they may combine features of the two consonants into a single sound, e.g., *swing* [fɪŋ], maintaining the frication of [s] and the labiality of [w]. Thus there are many ways of achieving the goal of cluster simplification. Which one (or ones) is used depends on the level of articulatory development (based in part on maturational factors) and on the cognitive strategies adopted by the child. To take an extreme case, a child who is unable to produce initial clusters may simply not try to say any words beginning with two consonants; such a solution to the "problem" of consonant clusters is obviously a cognitive one.

Although the various theoretical positions regarding universal patterns and individual differences may be reconciled, there are other differences that are not so easily resolved. Three of these are mentioned briefly. First is the issue of *linguistic perception*. Stampe claimed that perception is completely developed at the onset of meaningful speech. In contrast, Waterson as well as Macken and Ferguson argued that perception is still developing in the initial stages and that children may perceive adult words (or utterances) as unanalyzed units and only later as sequences of segments.

The second issue involves the *relationship of babbling and meaningful speech*. Jakobson stated explicitly that there is no relationship here—that babbling and speech represent two distinct periods of phonological development. In contrast, Locke postulated that the phonological patterns of first words are essentially identical to those of babbling, and Mowrer claimed that the babbling patterns are shaped through reinforcement so that they resemble more and more closely the patterns of adult speech. The other theories do not specifically address the relationship of babbling and speech, but seem to assume that they are closely related.

Finally, there is the issue of the *role of input*. Stampe claimed that input has little effect on acquisition, whereas Mowrer, Olmsted, and Waterson (and to a lesser extent Macken and Ferguson) believed that input plays a crucial role. However, they did not all agree on the nature of the relationship between input and phonological learning. With this issue and those cited earlier, empirical studies that test specific hypotheses are needed to evaluate the various theories.

In conclusion, it is clear that our current knowledge of phonological acquisition is not sufficient, from either a theoretical or an empirical point of view, for the formulation of a comprehensive model of development. However, we can begin to make some proposals regarding what that model should include. The basic components, described briefly below, are not independent phenomena but interact closely with one another:

1. **Auditory-perceptual component** Encompasses the ability to attend to and perceive linguistic input.
2. **Cognitive component** Encompasses the ability to recognize,

store, and retrieve input; to formulate rules for output; and to compare input and output.

3. **Phonological component** Encompasses the ability to use sounds contrastively and to match the phonological distinctions of the adult language.

4. **Neuromotor component** Encompasses the ability to plan and execute the articulatory movements underlying speech.

Although other components may also be necessary, we feel these, at the very least, are essential for any model of phonological development.

Chapter 4

Methodological Issues

The methods used in the collection and analysis of data play an important part in the study of phonological development. All too often researchers fail to give adequate attention to methodological issues, and consequently their results are weakened by the use of inappropriate techniques for gathering or analyzing the data. The purpose of this chapter is to describe methodologies currently used in the study of child phonology and to evaluate their strengths and weaknesses. Although the examples are drawn primarily from investigations of normally developing children, the methodological questions raised are also relevant to studies of children with disordered phonology. A discussion of the techniques most appropriate for clinical purposes appears in Chapter 6. The present chapter is divided into two major sections: the first is devoted to *data collection*, the second to *data analysis*.

Before we begin the discussion of various methodologies, it is important to point out that there is no single method for the collection or analysis of data that is appropriate for all types of studies. Decisions regarding sample size, the nature of the sample, and appropriate techniques for data analysis all depend on the goals of the particular investigation. For example, knowledge of the *process* of phonological acquisition is best gained through the study of a few children with data taken at frequent (daily or near-daily) intervals, whereas the establishment of age norms must be based on data from many children.

Data Collection

The primary issues related to data collection are: (1) number of subjects; (2) number and frequency of data collection sessions; (3) techniques for obtaining the speech sample; (4) size and nature of the corpus; and (5) methods of recording and transcribing the data. Each of these variables is discussed separately in the sections that follow even though in many cases they do not function independently of one another.

Subjects

The major variable regarding subjects is *sample size,* which can range from one to several hundred or more. Case studies of a single child (e.g., Labov and Labov, 1978; Smith, 1973) provide valuable in-depth accounts of phonological acquisition but are not appropriate as the basis for statements regarding general patterns of development. Conversely, large-sample investigations, of 40–400 or more, e.g., those of Templin (1947, 1957), are used for documenting group trends and determining age norms but tell us little about the specific details of each subject's phonological system. During the last decade there have been a number of small-group studies, of 2 to 8 subjects (e.g., Ferguson and Farwell, 1975; Stoel-Gammon and Cooper, 1981, 1984), designed to investigate individual differences in acquisition. To be valuable, such studies must include enough subjects to define the possible range of differences and at the same time enough detail on each subject to permit the identification of variation in the process of development.

Regardless of the sample size, researchers should be sure that their "normally developing" subjects are indeed normal by assessing their hearing acuity and ascertaining that their cognitive functioning is within the normal range. If the study involves subjects with sensory deficits or developmental delays, these should be described and documented as completely as is possible.

Longitudinal Versus Cross-sectional Data

Longitudinal studies trace the development of a given child or group of children over a period of time. In most cases data are collected at regular intervals ranging from the daily observations of some diary studies to semiannual or annual sessions. Longitudinal data allow the researcher to observe the patterns individual children follow in acquiring their phonological system.

Cross-sectional studies are based on data from a child or group of children at a single point in time. Data from a group of children at a given age are useful in that they provide information regarding the *norms* for that age. In some investigations researchers have used cross-sectional data from subject groups at specific ages as the basis for inferring longitudinal patterns of development (e.g., Templin, 1957; Wellman et al., 1931). Although age-related stages can be based on cross-sectional data, it cannot be assumed that individual children pass through each of these stages during the period of acquisition. Only *longitudinal* studies can provide information regarding the developmental stages of an individual child or group of children.

Although logically independent, the variables of sample size, longitudinal versus cross-sectional data, and frequency of data collection usually interact. Because of practical considerations, it is generally not feasible to carry out a longitudinal study of a large number of subjects in which data are collected at frequent (daily or weekly) intervals. In most investigations, there is a trade-off. If the sample size is large, data are collected only once (i.e., are cross-sectional) or at infrequent intervals (e.g., semiannually or annually). If the sample size is small, data are collected more frequently. Both types of investigation provide valuable information that leads to a better understanding of child phonology.

Collecting a Sample

One of the major variables in any investigation of phonological development is the way in which the data are gathered. Methods of data collection can be placed on a continuum with informal observational techniques at one end and formal, highly structured methods at the other. For those studies in which data collection is truly informal, vocal productions are not elicited but simply allowed to occur as part of the natural interaction between the subject and another person, often the caretaker, e.g., Labov and Labov's diary study (1978), or between the child and his or her environment, as in the crib monologues recorded by Weir (1962). The primary advantage of this mode of data collection is that the samples obtained are ecologically valid; they represent the child's spontaneous speech productions in a natural setting. The subjects vocalize when and as often as they wish; they interact naturally with the persons and objects around them; and, during the linguistic period, they produce the words, phrases, and sentences of their choice. However, there are some major disadvantages to this method: (1) data collection and data analysis are often very time-consuming, e.g., diary studies; (2) the samples may not include a sufficient number or variety of words or utterances to permit a thorough analysis, e.g., a given phoneme may not occur in all word positions needed for analysis; and (3) subject samples are often so different that it is difficult to make comparisons across subjects.

A slightly more formal method of data collection, which we call semistructured, attempts to maintain the advantages described above while eliminating the disadvantages. In these investigations (e.g., Macken and Barton's study of the acquisition of the voicing contrast, 1980), the setting remains informal with data collected in the home or in a home-like setting at a university or school. Subjects are encouraged to talk, but no direct elicitation measures are used. Typically, the experimenter introduces props, e.g., books or toys, in an effort to get the child to verbalize. These props are carefully selected so that the words produced by the child include the target phones needed for analysis. In Macken and Barton's (1980) study, for example, the stimuli were chosen to elicit words with initial stop consonants. The major advantages of this method of data collection are: (1) it is less time-consuming than the informal method described above because data collection occurs during a scheduled period, usually 30–60 min for each session; (2) it works well with young children in the earliest stages of linguistic development, around age 1;0–2;6; and (3) it provides the researcher with productions of words from a predetermined set of lexical items, thereby facilitating intersubject comparisons. Word productions are not identical across subjects, however, because most children produce only a subset of the desired words.

In the most structured type of data collection, the formal, highly structured method, the goal is to obtain a specified set of responses. Data are typically gathered in a formal setting in which the subject is requested to produce either spontaneously or in imitation a *predetermined set* of utterances, usually single words. In some studies, (e.g., Smith, 1978), the child is asked to imitate nonsense forms.

Elicitation Methods When formal data collection procedures are used, the speech sample is usually elicited in one of two ways: (1) *elicited naming*, in which the child is asked to name the object or action shown in a picture; or (2) *elicited imitation*, in which the child is asked to repeat a list of words produced by the experimenter. Other methods are also used, although not as frequently as those described above. These include *sentence completion* and *sentence recall*. In a sentence completion task, the experimenter describes a scene in a picture, and the child is asked to provide a key word in the description. For example, to elicit the word *fish,* the subject is shown a picture of a man catching a fish. The experimenter points to the picture and says something like "This is a man; this is a fish. The man is catching the _____." In most cases, the child finishes the sentence with the appropriate word (Ingram et al., 1980). In a sentence recall task, the subject is asked to describe a picture as the experimenter had described it. For the word *fish* in the previous example, the expected response would be "The man is catching the fish." In both sentence completion and sentence recall, the form produced by the child is a *deferred imitation* rather than a spontaneous production.

Particular attention should be given to the variable of method of elicitation because it may affect the child's pronunciation of a word. For spontaneous productions, the child must rely on his or her own underlying representation of the word, whereas in an imitation task the child must repeat the word modeled by the experimenter. If the word is already part of his productive vocabulary, the child has an underlying representation for that word; the pronunciation of the word may then be based on the child's underlying form *or* on the modeled form. However, if the word is not part of his vocabulary, the child has only the modeled form as the basis for his pronunciation. Consequently, a child's pronunciation of a target phoneme, or word, may be different in imitated and spontaneous production. The advantage of using *spontaneous naming,* then, is that the child's productions are more likely to be similar to utterances produced in a natural, nontest setting. The disadvantages are that elicitation of a list of names can be time-consuming, that some target words are difficult to represent using pictures, and that in some cases the child may not know the target word. The advantages and disadvantages of using *elicited imitations* represent the reverse side of the coin. Data collection is fast and not hampered by the subject's lack of familiarity with certain words; at the same time, the resultant productions are likely to be less representative of a child's pronunciation patterns in spontaneous speech.

It is often assumed that imitated words are more accurate than spontaneously produced words. However, the few studies that have examined this variable provide conflicting findings. A number of large-scale studies reported no differences between the two types of productions, including Templin's study (1947) of 100 subjects ages 2;0–6;0, Paynter and Bumpas' study (1977) of 100 subjects ages 3;0–3;6, and Ingram et al.'s study (1980) of initial fricatives, which included 73 children ages 1;10–5;11. In contrast, Siegel et al. (1963) reported that for their subjects, 100 kindergarten children (average age 5;4), articulation was significantly better in imitated responses on eight of the 40 sounds tested; Kersheck and Socolofsky (1972) also found differences in the responses of a group of 4-year-olds: 40 of the 45 subjects tested obtained better articulation scores in the production of imitated responses. Finally, Johnson and Somers (1978) tested two groups of British children, 32 "younger" subjects (mean age 4;9) and 32 "older" subjects (mean age 5;9) and found that mean articulation scores of both groups were higher in the imitative than in the spontaneous mode. Given these conflicting findings, no conclusive statements regarding the effect of imitation on pronunciation can be made.

Most of these studies have focused on the question: Are elicited imitations pronounced more accurately than spontaneous productions? In fact, the issue of differences due to mode of elicitation should be broader than this. It may be that there are no differences in the number of *correct* responses but that differences exist in the types of *errors* that occur in imitated and spontaneous production. For example, the interdental fricative /ð/ may be produced as [d] in spontaneous forms, e.g., *feather* [fɛdɚ] but as [v] or [z] in imitation (Moskowitz, 1975).

Moreover, there is another type of imitation that may affect pronunciation patterns: spontaneous—rather than elicited—imitation. For the purpose of this discussion, *spontaneous imitation* is defined as the child's repetition of part, or all, of an utterance produced by another speaker, e.g., Mom: "Look at the giraffe." Child (spontaneous imitation): "Giraffe." Although there is considerable individual variation in the amount of imitation, spontaneous imitations occur relatively frequently in children's speech between ages 1;0 and 3;0 (Bloom et al., 1974). As in the case of elicited imitations, the effects of spontaneous imitation on pronunciation are not well understood. There seems to be general agreement that imitated productions are often different from spontaneous ones, but the nature and extent of the differences have not been well documented. Waterson (1971) studied her son's early speech development and reported that spontaneous imitations were often produced with greater phonetic accuracy than nonimitated forms. Shibamoto and Olmsted (1978) found that spontaneously imitated words, although not necessarily more accurate than spontaneous productions, often introduced phonological forms (either phones or syllabic structures) that did not occur in their subject's spontaneous output. Clumeck (1977) found that his Chinese-learning subject also produced a wider range of speech sounds in imitated forms but noted that both imitated and spontaneous speech "appeared to be subject to the same general constraints, and when a change took place in the imitated speech, it would often show up in spontaneous speech as well."

Given the differences that have been observed in the two types of speech, it is best to note whether an utterance was produced spontaneously or as an imitation and then to analyze the two sets of utterances independently. In this way, the extent and nature of the differences can be determined.

The Corpus

As with the other variables discussed so far, the size and nature of the corpus depends on the goals of the investigation. If the research is directed toward variability in pronunciation of the stressed vowel /o/, renditions of /o/ in 15–20 words may provide the desired information; or if the study focuses on the acquisition of prevocalic liquids, the corpus should include only those words with /l/ or /r/ in prevocalic position. For the discussion that follows, it is assumed that the goal is to assess a child's phonological system by analyzing productions of all the phonemes of English in all word positions. Even when the goal is as narrowly defined as this, there are a number of variables that must be considered. The most important of these are discussed below.

Single Words Versus Continuous Speech A major consideration is whether to gather a sample of single-word productions obtained through spontaneous naming or imitation tasks, or to use a corpus of continuous speech obtained through naturally occurring conversational interactions or through story-telling.

The advantages of a single-word assessment procedure are that it is relatively fast, and the word list obtained can be designed to ensure that all the phonemes are tested in specific word pictures. Moreover, the single-word-naming task can be administered to a group of children, thus providing comparable data sets across children. Finally, the task can be readministered at a later date to assess a child's progress over time.

A serious disadvantage of a single-word assessment procedure is that it does not give a complete picture of a child's phonological abilities, because it provides no data on pronunciation patterns as they occur in a natural communicative setting, i.e., continuous speech. Clearly, the task of naming single words requires different skills than the sequencing of words in phrases or sentences with syntactic and semantic structure. Thus it is not surprising that the few investigations that have compared the pronunciation patterns evident in single-word productions with those of running speech in the same groups of subjects have reported finding differences in the two types of data (Bank et al., 1983; Dubois and Bernthal, 1978; Shriberg and Kwiatkowski, 1980).

The advantage of using continuous speech, then, is that it is representative of a child's speech patterns. However, there are some disadvantages. First, it is more time-consuming (and often more difficult) to phonetically transcribe continuous speech than single-word productions. Second, even when the speech sample is fairly long (80–100 utterances), the range of target phonemes and vocabulary items attempted by the child may be quite restricted. Finally, if the child's speech is highly unintelligible, it is difficult to determine the adult words that were attempted, thus making it impossible to compare the child's productions with the adult model. If a continuous-speech sample is used, it must be remembered that words may be pronounced differently in casual speech than in more formal settings. For example, the phrases, *What's that* and *Can you* are often produced as [wʌtsæʔ] and [kjū], respectively, in natural conversational interactions (Stoel-Gammon, 1983b). Such productions should not be analyzed as incorrect when they occur as part of a continuous-speech sample.

Target Words Another consideration when using a single word assessment task involves the *words* the child is asked to produce. Ideally, the word list would contain all the target phonemes of English as singleton phonemes, and in clusters and diphthongs. The phonemes should appear in various word positions, including word initial, medial, and final.

For a thorough assessment, each phoneme should be produced several times in each word position. As was shown in the previous chapter, pronunciation of a target phoneme can vary considerably during the period of mastery, either in multiple renditions of a single word, e.g., *sun* pronounced as [dʌn] or [tʃʌn], or across words, e.g., /d/ is [d] in *doll* and *door* but [g] in *duck* and *dog* (due to Velar Assimilation). Thus, analyzing a child's phonological system on the basis of a single production of each phoneme does not provide a truly representative assessment of his or her abilities.

Phoneme production is not only subject to intra- and inter-word variation, it is also affected by such factors as word length and the child's familiarity with the word (Wellman et al., 1931). In their study of initial fricatives, Ingram and his colleagues (1980) found that, on the average, the proportion of correct productions was higher in monosyllabic, commonly used words (e.g., *fish, vase,* and *zees*) than in longer, less common forms (e.g., *farina, volcano,* and *zucchini*). The relationship did not hold true for all forms, however; the phoneme /θ-/ was pronounced correctly more often in the word *thermometer* than in the shorter word *thief*. In sum, it is obvious that testing a phoneme in just one word cannot provide a representative sample of a child's phonological system.

Size of the Sample The number of words or utterances that should be included in a corpus depends, in part, on the stage of development of the child. As noted above, ideally each target sound is assessed in multiple renditions of the same word and in a variety of target words of differing lengths and phonetic configurations. If each phoneme is assessed in this manner, the resulting corpus will contain 250–300 words or utterances, and data collection, transcription, and analysis will be lengthy.

One way to shorten the procedure is to collect a preliminary sample of 75–100 words or utterances to check the child's level of mastery and extent of variability. If the preliminary corpus reveals that stops and nasals exhibit little variability, for example, and are usually produced correctly, the focus of the assessment should be directed toward productions of phonemes that are still unstable: fricatives, affricates, and liquids. Productions of these sound classes should be obtained in a variety of words.

Recording and Transcribing Data

An important methodological consideration for any investigation of child speech is the recording and transcription of the data obtained. Not all studies use audio recordings of the data. In most diary studies, for example, the child's utterances are transcribed phonetically on site, and in many articulation tests productions are not tape-recorded; rather, the target phoneme is transcribed or coded "correct" or "incorrect" on a special coding sheet. One advantage of on-site coding is that the transcriber can note oral and facial movements, e.g., lip rounding or tongue protrusion, that may affect articulation of a target sound. A second advantage is that there is no need for a microphone or other recording equipment, which may be intimidating for a child. Finally, on-site transcription takes relatively little time. In spite of these advantages, there is a serious disadvantage: because the data are not recorded, there is no way to check the accuracy of on-site transcriptions.

The amount of detail that should be included in a phonetic transcription depends entirely on the purpose of the study. If the aim is to determine which phonemes are produced correctly and which are not, the level of transcription can be quite broad. However, if the goal is to describe correct and incorrect productions in some detail, the transcription should be quite narrow and include diacritical markings and segmental phones not found in the adult language. A chart of the phonetic symbols and diacritics appropriate for a narrow phonetic transcription is presented in Appendix A.

Although phonetic transcriptions are usually considered to be a means of *recording* the pronunciation of a word or phrase, they are, in fact, a form of *analysis*. As Strange and Broen (1980) noted: "It is not possible to have a transcription system that is free from the effects of (the transcriber's) phonological theory." Researchers (and clinicians) should be aware that the transcription system they adopt will influence data analysis and may also affect the results of their study (Allen, 1977).

Summary

In sum, all the variables discussed above need to be considered in selecting phonological data. Although they were described independently, the factors interact in predictable ways, and these interactions should also be taken into account. For example, if a child's speech is to be transcribed narrowly, with much detail, the recording equipment should be of very high quality and the sample obtained in a quiet setting, ideally a sound-treated room. If, on the other hand, a broader transcription is used, the quality of recording equipment and the setting are not so important. Decisions regarding data collection not only affect the quality and nature of the corpus but also the data analysis, as is seen in the following section.

Data Analysis

As with data collection, the appropriate methodology for data analysis depends on the goals of the particular study in question. Most investigations of child phonology have been *perceptually based* (i.e., based on phonetically transcribed data); perceptually based analyses are most appropriate when the goal is to identify and describe overall *patterns* of correct and incorrect productions. Such analyses are limited in certain respects, however, because they depend entirely on the auditory-perceptual capabilities of the transcriber(s) and, as was mentioned in the previous section, they are affected by biases introduced by the transcription system itself.

Throughout the discussion, it is assumed that the goal of our analysis is to describe an entire phonological system, not some portion of it. For such an analysis, transcription-based investigations are a necessity. In some cases, however, instrumental (or acoustic) analyses may be used to supplement the transcription in order to study certain aspects of speech production that are difficult to transcribe reliably. Such aspects include voice onset time (e.g., Maxwell and Weismer, 1982), segment duration (e.g., Smith, 1978), vowel quality (e.g., Liberman, 1980), and fundamental frequency (e.g., Menn, 1976b).

Various techniques for analyzing child speech are presented first, along with a discussion of some of the problems involved. Then the techniques are illustrated in detailed analyses of speech samples from two children.

Techniques for Analyzing Child Speech

Although the basic goals are similar, applying the techniques of phonological analysis used for adult languges to the production of a single child or a group of children is not as straightforward as it might seem. It was stated in Chapter 1 that the goal of a phonological analysis is to determine the inventory of contrastive units, or phonemes, that occur in a language and then to describe their patterns of occurrence.

In adult speech, phonemes can be identified because they exhibit consistent behaviors across words. In the early stages of child speech, however, production of a phonemic target may vary considerably from word to word, often making it impossible to determine the inventory of phonemes and phonemic contrasts. It has been suggested that the contrastive unit at this stage of development is the *word* or perhaps the *syllable* rather than the phoneme (Ferguson and Farwell, 1975; Menyuk and Menn, 1979). Consequently, analysis of a child's early words in terms of adult-based phonemes may provide only a confusing picture of seemingly random behavior, whereas a word-based analysis reveals consistent patterns based on word length, syllable shape, and/or permitted sound sequences (Macken, 1979).

In the later stages, when the productions can be analyzed in terms of adult-like phonemes, the presence of phonetic variability makes a traditional phonological analysis more difficult. Whereas the adult phonological system is relatively stable, the child's system is in a constant state of change with new phones and new forms entering the repertoire while older forms disappear. Because the acquisition process occurs gradually, new and old forms often coincide for a period, giving rise to extensive variability both within and across words. This variability is increased by the presence of *frozen forms*, i.e., pronunciations that remain unchanged when the rest of the phonology improves, and *advanced forms*, i.e., words whose pronunciation is more accurate than would be expected.

Variability is not the only problem in attempting to perform a traditional phonemic analysis. Even when children's speech patterns are relatively stable, there are aspects of production that are difficult to describe using conventional forms of analysis. For example, if a child produces the phoneme /s/ correctly in final position but always substitutes [t] for adult /s/ in initial position and [z] for /s/ intervocalically, can we say that [s] is a phoneme in the child's system? Clearly, in final position, *s* is a contrastive sound segment that behaves like a phoneme, but in other word positions, there is no evidence that [s] is phonemic. The most accurate way to describe the behavior of [s], then, is in terms of word position; it is contrastive in final position but not in other positions.

Types of Analysis

The following sections present a discussion of current techniques used in phonological analysis of child speech and provide examples based on two sets of data. As stated earlier, the appropriate methods of analysis are determined by the goals of the study in question. Throughout the discussion that follows, it is assumed that the goal is to provide a general description of a child's phonological system in terms of the inventory of phones produced, positional and sequential constraints on the production of phones, contrastive units present in the child's speech, and similarities and differences between the child's system and the adult system. The phonological samples analyzed are from children beyond the very early stages of production, and thus the contrastive units mentioned above are phonemes rather than words or syllables.

There are two major types of analysis used in describing a child's phonological system: one describes the child's production without reference to the adult model, and the other compares the child's pronunciation with the adult form of the word. Analysis of the child's productions as a self-contained system, referred to as *independent analysis,* includes the following: (1) an inventory of phones classified by word position and articulatory features; (2) an inventory of syllable and word shapes produced; and (3) sequential constraints on the occurrence of phones.

In the second type of analysis, referred to as *relational analysis,* the adult form and the child's pronunciation are compared. Patterned, or systematic, differences are then described in terms of sound segments, features, rules, or phonological processes, or a combination of these. The particular form of analysis depends on the purpose of the study; in the analysis presented in the following sections, for example, the correspondence between the adult and child form are described using sound segments, features, and processes.

Relational analyses not only reveal how closely the child's pronunciations match the adult's, but also serve as the basis for comparing the child's emerging *phonemic* system with the adult system. There are two basic types of correspondences: those in which the phonemic contrasts of the adult system are maintained in the child's productions and those in which the contrasts are lost.

Examples of adult–child correspondences that *maintain* phonemic contrasts include: (1) cases in which the child's pronunciation of the target phonemes matches the adult model, e.g., /s/ and /ʃ/ contrast when both are pronounced correctly; and (2) cases in which the child's pronunciation of a target phoneme differs *phonetically* from the adult phoneme but is a distinctive sound segment (i.e., a phoneme) within the child's system, e.g., adult /ʃ/ is pronounced as a lateral fricative [ɬ], thus maintaining the contrast between /s/ and /ʃ/.

Examples of segmental correspondences resulting in the *loss* of a phonemic contrast include: (1) cases in which two adult phonemes are rendered as a single phone by the child, e.g., adult /s/ and /ʃ/ are produced [s]; (2) cases in which a single adult phoneme is rendered variably as two (or more) phones, and in the adult system these phones represent contrastive phonemes, e.g., adult /ʃ/ is pronounced either [s] or [ʃ]; and (3) cases in which an adult phoneme is omitted. The last pattern typically occurs in specific word positions or phonetic contexts, e.g., at the end of words— *buy* [baɪ] versus *bite* [baɪ]—and in consonant clusters—*no* [no] versus *snow* [no].

Caveats

Two issues related to adult–child analyses need to be discussed before moving on to some sample analyses. Adult–child comparisons are typically displayed as *dog* [gɔg], *rope* [wop], or *ball* [ba], and it seems to be assumed that the adult form of a word is pronounced the same by all speakers and in all linguistic contexts. In reality, this is not the case; it has been well documented that the pronunciation of words and phonemes may vary from speaker to speaker because of age or sex differences and regional and social variation (Bright, 1976). Even if the target forms are based on data from a single speaker, variation may occur owing to differences in *speech style*, e.g., slow careful speech versus rapid colloquial speech (Stoel-Gammon, 1983b). Thus it must be understood that when a child's pronunciation is compared with the "adult model" the comparison is based on an *idealized* target form that in reality represents only one possible pronunciation of the word (Locke, 1981; Smith, 1979).

The second issue deals with two beliefs regarding the child's production, i.e., that: (1) children perceive and encode adult words in an adult-like manner (Smith, 1973; Stampe, 1969); and (2) they then attempt to pronounce the words correctly. Neither of these assumptions can be taken for granted. Although phonemic perception is not fully understood, there is evidence from a number of studies that the perception and encoding of words is not always adult-like during the period of phonological development (Garnica, 1973; Kornfeld, 1971). Consequently, a child's mispronunciations may be due to perceptual errors or production errors (see Chapter 3). If the errors are indeed production errors, another problem arises: How does one determine if the child tried to produce the articulatory targets but failed, or if he or she simply attempted to achieve an *acoustic approximation* of the adult word. Whereas some production errors are due to motoric difficulties, others may be attributed to organizational and production constraints that simplify the adult form *before* it is articulated (Ferguson, 1978; Ingram, 1976; Menn, 1980). Thus it cannot simply be assumed that a child always attempts to produce an accurate rendition of adult words. If these limitations are kept in mind, adult–child comparisons provide a valuable framework for describing a child's phonological system.

The remainder of the chapter provides sample analyses of the speech of two normally developing children, ages 2;2 and 3;5. Because of differences in level of development, slightly different analysis procedures are used for the two samples. In both cases, however, the subjects' productions are first analyzed in terms of the child's system, then in terms of an adult–child comparison.

Sample I: SR, Age 2;2

The productions in this sample are from a girl, SR, who was age 2;2 at the time of data collection. The sample consists of 75 words and a total of 88 productions as a result of multiple renditions of some items. The words, presented in Table 4.1, were selected from a larger corpus of utterances produced during a play session. The *independent analysis*, presented first, includes three parts: (1) an inventory of phones; (2) an inventory of syllable and word shapes with frequency of occurrence; and (3) statements regarding sequential constraints on the occurrence of phones.

Table 4.1 SR Age 2;2: 75 Selected Words

Gloss	Transcription	Gloss	Transcription	Gloss	Transcription
all-done	'dada	hat	ʔæt	sock	gak
alone	wõn	hi	haɪ, aɪ	spill	pʰiṵ, biṵ
around	waõn	hot	ʔat	splash	pʰæs, bæs
asleep	jip	jar	da	spoon	pʰũn, bũn
ball	ba	jello	'dɛwo	stop	dap, tʰap
banana	'nænə	jelly	'dɛji	table	'tʰebu
big	bɪk	juice	du, dus	teeth	tʰif, tʰi
blanket	'babi	king	kʰĩŋ	thank-you	'gæku
block	bak, gak	laugh	wæf	there	dɛ
bottle	'badu	leave	jif	these	dis
bridge	bɪtṣ	little	'jɪdu	throw	tʰo, do
brush	bʌs	look	wʊk	tickle	'gɪku
butter	'bʌdu	mommy	'mami	tomato	'medo
car	kʰa	nice	naɪ	tooth	tʰuf, duf
chair	tʰɛ, dɛ	nothing	'nʌfɪŋ	touch	dʌtṣ, tʰʌtṣ
cheese	tʰi, tʰis	pajama	'dæmə	trouble	'dʌbu
chicken	'gɪkə̃n	peach	pʰitṣ	truck	gʌk
dish	dɪs	pedal	'bɛdu	van	bæn
doggie	'gɔgi	popcorn	'gakõn	very	'bɛwi
duck	gʌk	return	tʰũn	wash	was
feet	pʰit	ride	waɪt	wheel	wiṵ
fork	pʰɔk	room	wũm	with	wɪf
giraffe	wæf	school	kʰu	zebra	'dibwə
good	gʊt	seven	'dɛbən	zipper	'dɪpu
hand	hæn	shirt	dʊt	zoo	du

Independent Analysis

Phonetic Inventory: Distribution and Articulatory Features The phonetic inventory (Table 4.2) shows all the phones occurring in SR's productions, grouped according to their position in the word and classified by manner of articulation. Phones occurring once or twice are marked by parentheses and should be considered marginal in the analysis. The table also includes consonant clusters.

When the data are displayed in this way, certain patterns of occurrence become evident in SR's data:

1. Although the inventory includes a full range of stop, nasal, and glide consonants, the number of fricatives and affricates is severely limited (only [f, s, t͜s] occur), and there are no instances of liquid phones.
2. Fricatives and affricates occur with some frequency in final position (in more than 15 words), only marginally in medial position (just one word), and never in initial position.
3. All oral consonants (i.e., stops and fricatives) in final position are voiceless; in initial and medial position, both voiced and voiceless phones occur.

Table 4.2 Phonetic Inventory: Initial, Medial, and Final Position

	Word Position		
Manner	**Initial**	**Medial**	**Final**
Stop	p^h	(p)^a	p
	b	b	
	t^h		t
	d	d	
	(k^h)	k	k
	g	(g)	
	(ʔ)		
Fricative/affricate		(f)	f
			s
			t͜s
Nasal	(m)	(m)	(m)
	n	n	n
			(ŋ)
Glide	w	w	
	j	(j)	
	(h)		
Cluster		bw	

^aSounds that occurred fewer than three times are noted in parentheses.

Syllable and Word Shapes The word shapes produced by SR are described in terms of their C (consonant) and V (vowel or diphthong) structures along with the number of occurrences of each word shape. These numbers are useful in determining which forms are well established in the child's system.

Word shapes	Number of Occurrences
V	1
CV	15
CVC	39
'CVCV	19
'CVCCV	1
'CVCVC	4

This analysis reveals that SR's words have a relatively simple structure; they are either monosyllables, primarily CV or CVC, or disyllables with stress on the first syllable. Such forms are typical of a child age 2;0–2;6. The only occurrence of a consonant cluster (in *zebra* [dibwə]) should be regarded as a marginal form in SR's system.

In terms of *syllable* shapes, SR's productions included an overwhelming proportion of CV and CVC syllables. There is one example of a vowel alone (V) and one instance of a consonant cluster (CCV). All other syllables are CV or CVC.

Sequential Constraints Although there are several positional constraints on the occurrence of phones (see Table 4.2), there seem to be only two sequential constraints: (1) except for the lone occurrence of [bw] in *zebra,* there are no sequences of consonants; (2) when the second consonant of a CVC sequence is a velar, the first is never an alveolar or a palatal; this constraint holds even if the CVC sequence is embedded in a longer string of phones, e.g., *chicken* [gɪkən], *tickle* [gɪku].

It is always difficult to make decisive statements regarding phonetic and syllabic inventories and sequential constraints in any child's corpus without reference to the adult pronunciation. If the corpus contains no tokens of the phone [r] in initial and [f] in final position, for example, there are two possible causes. The child may be omitting these sounds or substituting other sounds when attempting to produce words that begin with /r/ or end with /f/. An alternative explanation to the observed pattern is that the child's corpus contains no words beginning with /r/ or ending with /f/. If this is the case, the distributional pattern is due to insufficient data rather than to lack of development of the child's phonological system. The problem of describing *sequential constraints* is even thornier, because even a very large corpus does not contain tokens of all possible sequences. For example, in the above corpus the segment [m] occurs only twice as the initial consonant of a word—in the sequence [mami] (*mommy*) and [medo] (*tomato*). Are we to conclude that there is a constraint on the production of initial [m] in all other phonetic environments? Presumably not, but the data on hand seem to support such a constraint.

It is clear from the examples above that an "independent" analysis must in fact refer in part to the adult words in the corpus. Although the child's pronunciations are not compared directly with the adult form, knowledge of the adult words allows us to determine which sound and sound sequences are to be expected. In the above corpus, for example, alveolar stops occur in a variety of phonetic contexts in the adult words, whereas in the child's productions the contexts are far more restricted. In sum, although referred to as being independent, this first type of analysis must take into consideration some aspects of the adult utterances the child is trying to produce.

Relational Analysis

The second analysis is a comparison of SR's production with the (idealized) adult form of the words. The comparisons are first described in terms of phonological processes and natural classes based on distinctive features. Then the adult phonemic system is compared with that of the child.

Phonological Process Analysis Using the phonological processes defined in Chapter 2, the following processes are evident in SR's data. These processes are summarized at the end of this section.

1. **Unstressed Syllable Deletion** All adult words beginning with an unstressed syllable were produced with omission of that syllable:

alone	won	giraffe	wæf
around	waʊn	pajama	dæmə
asleep	jip	return	tʊn
banana	nænə	tomato	medo

2. **Final Consonant Deletion** The process of final consonant deletion occurred infrequently and may be disappearing from SR's system. It applied consistently to final liquids and inconsistently to final fricatives:

ball	ba	juice	du, dus
car	ka	nice	naɪ
cheese	ti, tis	school	ku

Although final nasals and stops were not deleted in other words, the final consonants of *all-done* (pronounced [dada]) and *blanket* ([babi]) were deleted. These forms are more primitive than would be expected in light of SR's other pronunciations and may be *frozen forms* (see below).

3. **Stopping**   Stopping occurred without exception in initial position, affecting 20 words in the sample; there is one example in medial position (of two possible occurrences) and none in word-final position (of 16 possible occurrences). Some examples of the process include:

jello	'dɛwo	sock	gak
fork	pok	these	dis
shirt	dʊt	very	'bɛwi

4. **Depalatalization**   In initial position, palatal fricatives and affricates were produced as stops, as shown above. In final position, the manner of production remains unchanged but they are *depalatalized* and produced as alveolar fricatives and affricates:

bridge	bɪts̪	splash	pæs, bæs
brush	bʌs	touch	tʌts̪, dʌts̪
dish	dɪs	wash	was

5. **Gliding of Liquids**   In all instances, prevocalic liquids /l, r/ were substituted by glides, /r/ by [w] and /l/ by [j] or [w]:

giraffe	wæf	jello	'dɛwo
ride	waɪt	jelly	'dɛji
room	wum	laugh	wæf
very	'bɛwi	leave	jif
		little	'jɪdu
		look	wʊk

Examination of the substitutions for prevocalic /l/ reveals that [w] and [j] do not occur randomly but are determined by phonetic context. If the vowel that follows is a high front vowel, i.e., [i, ɪ], the substitute is [j]; for all other vowels, the substitute is [w].

6. **Vocalization**   In word-final position, syllabic liquids are produced as vowels:

bottle	'badu	table	'tebu
butter	'bʌdu	tickle	'gɪku
little	'jɪdu	trouble	'dʌbu

In two words, final /l/ is also produced as a vowel:

| spill | piṵ, biṵ |
| wheel | wiṵ |

7. **Cluster Reduction**   All target clusters, with the exception of the medial cluster in *zebra,* were reduced to a single consonant. The patterns of cluster reduction are generally those described in Chapter 2.

In clusters composed of /s + stop/, the /s/ is deleted; in SR's data, the remaining stop is either voiced or voiceless, unaspirated, e.g.:

| school | ku | spoon | pun, bun |
| spill | piṵ, biṵ | stop | tap, dap |

The only word in the sample containing a cluster composed of /s + liquid/ is *asleep;* here too the /s/ is deleted.

In clusters composed of /stop + liquid/, /liquid + stop/, or /liquid + nasal/, the liquid is always deleted. Some examples from SR's productions are:

bridge	bɪts̬	shirt	dʊt
fork	pok	throw	to, do
return	tʊn	trouble	'dʌbu

In clusters composed of /nasal + voiced stop/ the stop is deleted, but when the cluster is /nasal + voiceless stop/ the nasal is deleted:

| hand | hæn | thank you | 'gæku |
| around | waun | | |

However, more examples are needed to determine if this pattern occurs regularly.

8. **Voicing of Prevocalic Consonants**   Voiceless consonants in initial position are voiced in approximately half the target words produced by SR; in other words, voiceless targets remain voiceless or evidence variation in voicing:

pedal	'bɛdu	throw	to, do
seven	'dɛbən	tooth	tuf, duf
shirt	dʊt	touch	dʌts̬, tʌts̬

These data suggest that the voicing distinction in initial position is just becoming established in SR's system.

9. **Devoicing of Final Consonants**   All voiced obstruents (i.e., stops, fricatives, affricates) are produced as voiceless consonants in word-final position:

big	bɪk	leave	jif
bridge	bɪts̬	ride	waɪt
cheese	tis		

10. **Velar Assimilation**   SR's productions evidenced a pattern of *regressive* velar assimilation in which medial and final velar stops affected nonlabial consonants in initial position. The process occurred in all possible target words, e.g.:

chicken	'gɪkən	thank you	'gæku
doggie	'gɔgi	tickle	'gɪku
duck	gʌk	truck	gʌk

In addition, labial consonants were affected in two words (in one, the process was optional) but not in two others:

block	bak, gak	big	bɪk
popcorn	'gakon	fork	pok

11. **Sound Substitutions**   A few error patterns in SR's production affected only a single sound and thus cannot be considered general phonological processes. The sounds affected are shown below:

a. Target /θ/ is produced as [f]:

nothing	'nʌfɪŋ	tooth	tuf, duf
with	wɪf	teeth	tif

b. /h/ is optionally deleted or substituted by [ʔ]; in some words it is produced correctly:

hand	hæn	hi	haɪ, aɪ
hat	ʔæt	hot	ʔat

Idiosyncratic Forms   As mentioned above, there are two words in the sample that seem more primitive than the rest of SR's productions: *blanket* [babi] and *all-done* [dada]. Both appear to be frozen forms, although this hypothesis can only be verified through data from earlier stages of development.

In sum, this analysis provides evidence of 10 phonological

Table 4.3 Summary of Phonological Processes and Sound Substitutions

Process	Distributional Patterns
Unstressed Syllable Deletion	Initial syllables
Final Consonant Deletion	Liquids
	Fricatives
Stopping of fricatives and affricates	Initial position
Depalatalization	Final position
Gliding of liquids	Prevocalic position
Vocalization	Final syllabic liquids
	Final /l/ (nonsyllabic)
Cluster Reduction	All positions
Voicing of unvoiced consonants	Initial position
Devoicing of voiced consonants	Final position, non-nasal C
Velar assimilation	Regressive assimilation
Sound substitutions	θ → f
	h → ø,ʔ

processes and two sound substitutions in SR's system; except for Cluster Reduction, the processes are limited to specific word positions or to sound classes defined by articulatory features. The processes used by SR and their patterns of occurrence are summarized in Table 4.3.

Comparison of Phonemic Systems The extensive use of phonological processes in SR's productions results in the loss of many phonemic contrasts that occur in the adult language. In initial position, for example, contrasts between the following sounds or sound classes are lacking:

1. Between stops, fricatives, and affricates (due to the process of Stopping)
2. Between liquids and glides (due to the process of Gliding)
3. Between singleton consonants and consonant clusters (due to Cluster Reduction)

In addition, the contrast between voiced and voiceless consonants occurs only sporadically and is not well established.

In final position, contrasts that are not present in SR's system include:

1. The contrast between words ending in liquids and those ending in a vowel (due to deletion of final liquids)
2. The contrast between alveolar and palatal fricatives (due to Depalatalization)
3. The contrast between voiced and voiceless consonants (due to Final Consonant Devoicing)

These lists of contrasts are not meant to be exhaustive but are presented to demonstrate how phonological process analysis can be used to compare the adult phonemic system with that of the child.

Although the perception-based analysis shows that SR failed to produce contrasts between certain sound classes (e.g., stops and fricatives in initial position, voiced and voiceless consonants word finally), it is possible, at least in some cases, that phonemic distinctions are systematically maintained but are so slight as to be imperceptible to the transcriber. In such cases, acoustic analyses are needed to identify the presence of a contrast. For example, instrumental measurements of vowel duration might show that vowels preceding final voiced consonants (in the adult form) are longer than those preceding voiceless consonants or that renditions of initial [t] and [d] that serve as substitutes of /tʃ/ and /dʒ/, respectively, are longer than productions of [t] and [d] in words beginning with /t/ and /d/ in the adult form.

Although acoustic analyses may be desirable in some cases, they have two major drawbacks. First, they are very time consuming, and second, they require a fairly large number of examples to be reliable—ideally at least 20–25 words for each potential contrast. Thus, to determine if SR's renditions of stops differ from affricates, her corpus should contain 10 or more words beginning with /t/ and /d/ and the same number beginning with /tʃ/ and /dʒ/. In the present sample, and in many others, there simply are not enough examples for a reliable acoustic analysis.

Summary

It is clear from the various analyses presented above that SR's productions are quite primitive at this point in her development. She uses only a limited number of syllable types and word shapes, and a limited number of sound classes; moreover, the restrictions on the distribution of sounds are quite severe. Except for a few sound substitutions, the majority of errors can be described by phonological processes commonly found in the speech of children between ages 2;0 and 3;0. Her phonological system, although limited, is quite typical of children her age. If she continues to develop normally, her system will be much more adult-like in 12–15 months. As shown in the example from AJ, presented below, the phonological system of an older child contains a more extensive repertoire of word shapes and sound segments and many fewer restrictions on occurrence.

Table 4.4 AJ, Age 3:5: 93 Selected Words

Gloss	Transcription	Gloss	Transcription
another	əˈnʌdə	nice	naɪs
around	əˈwaʊnd	nobody	ˈnobaɾi
badge	bæʤ	nose	noːz
bathtub	ˈbæftʰʌb	nothing	ˈnʌfĩŋ
blood	blʌd	once	wʌnts
brother	ˈbwʌdə	pail	pʰeu̯
brush	bwʌʂ	pajamas	pʰəˈʤæməz
building	ˈbiu̯dĩŋ	play	plei, pəlei
carry	ˈkʰɛwi	push	puʂ
catch	kʰætʃ	riddle	ˈwɪdu
chair	tʃɛœ, tʃɛ	run	wʌn
cherries	ˈtʃɛwiz	rush	wʌʂ
chin	tʃĩn	scared	skɛːd
Christmas	ˈkwɪsməs	sell	sɛu̯
crash	kwæʂ	shelf	ʃɛu̯f
dinosaur	ˈdãɪnəsoə	ship	ʃɪp
door	dowə	shower	ˈʃauwə
drink	dwĩŋk	smart	smaːt
fall	fau̯	smell	smɛu̯
fish	fiʂ	snip	snɪp
five	faɪv	sorry	ˈsawi
flag	flæg, fəlæg	spill	spɪu̯
friend	fwẽnd	stamp	stæmp
galoshes	gəˈlaʂəz	stripe	stwaɪp
garage	gəˈwaʤ	sugar	ˈʃʊgə
giraffe	ʤəˈwæf	table	ˈtʰebu
give	gɪv	teeth	tʰif
glass	glæs	them	dɛ̃m
glove	glʌv, gəlʌv	think	fĩŋk
grass	gwæs	this	dɪs
gun	gʌn	thought	fat
handle	ˈhændu	three	fwi
heavy	ˈhɛvi	tickle	ˈtʰɪku
house	haus	Tinkerbell	ˈtʰĩŋkəbɛu̯
hungry	ˈhʌ̃ŋgwi	trick	twɪk
jar	ʤaœ, ʤa	tug	tʰʌg
jelly beans	ˈʤɛlibĩnz	velvet	ˈvɛu̯vət
jump	ʤʌmp	very	ˈvɛwi
library	ˈlaɪbwɛwi	watch	watʃ
like	laɪk	wishing	ˈwɪʂĩŋ
listen	ˈlɪsə̃n	with	wif
little	ˈlɪɾu	yard	jaːd
longer	ˈlãŋgə	yellow	ˈjɛlo
milk	mɪu̯k	zebra	ˈzibwə
more	mɔ	zipper	ˈzɪpʰœ
mouth	mauf	zoom	zũm
motorcycle	ˈmoɾəsaɪku		

Sample II: AJ, Age 3;5

The words in this sample were produced in a conversational set-ting by a boy, AJ, who was 3;5 at the time of data collection. As in the previous sample, the words appearing in the analysis were selected for illustrative purposes from a larger corpus of utter-ances. The corpus to be analyzed, presented in Table 4.4, contains 93 words and 98 utterances (because some words are included twice). The first analysis is of the child's productions without ref-erences to the adult model; the second is a comparison of the adult and child pronunciation.

Independent Analysis

Phonetic Inventory: Distribution and Articulatory Features
Initial and final phones in AJ's productions are shown in Table 4.5. (Medial phones are not considered in this illustrative analysis.) To be included, the phone must have occurred at least twice as the initial or final consonant. The phones are grouped according to their articulatory features of place and manner of production. Initial and final consonant clusters are also shown in the table. It can be seen from the table that AJ has an extensive repertoire of sound segments in terms of manner class (six classes of English

Table 4.5 Phonetic Inventory: Initial and Final Positions[a]

| | Inventory by Place of Articulation | | | | | | |
Manner	Labial	Labio-dental	Dental	Alveolar	Palatal	Velar	Glottal
Stop	p			t		k	
	b			d		g	
Fricative		f	-ṣ	s	ʃ-		
		v		z	ʒ		
Affricate					tʃ		
					ʤ		
Nasal	m			n		ŋ	
Liquid				l-			
Glide	w-				j-		h-

Clusters:
  Initial: bw-, fw-, dw-, kw-, gw-, pl-, bl-, fl-, gl-, sm-, sp-, sn-, st-, stw-, sk-.
  Final: -mp, -nts, -nd, -nz, -ŋk.

[a]Segments occurring in initial and final positions are listed without dashes. If a sound was restricted to one position, a dash indicates the position of occurrence (e.g., ʃ- indicates initial position only).

are represented) and place of articulation (phones occur at seven distinct places of articulation). Restrictions on the distribution of segments affect three phones: (1) dental [s̪] (a phone *not* found in adult English) occurs only in final position; (2) palatal [ʃ] occurs only word initially; and (3) liquid [l] occurs only in initial position.

Syllable and Word Shapes AJ uses a variety of syllable and word shapes including open and closed syllables and initial, medial, and final consonant clusters. Nine syllable types occur in the same sample: V, CV, CCV, CVC, CCVC, CVCC, CVCCC, CCVCC, and CCCVC. These syllable types are combined to form at least 20 word shapes ranging from the simple CV of *jar* [dʒa], to the relatively complex disyllable CCVC,CVC of the word *Christmas* [ˈkwɪsməs], to the trisyllabic shape CV,CCV,CV of *library* [ˈlaɪbwɛwi]. Overall, the most common word shapes are CVC and CVCV.

Sequential Constraints The sequential constraints evident in AJ's productions occur in the production of consonant clusters. In initial clusters composed of two members, if the first consonant is a stop or a nonsibilant fricative, the second member must be [w] or [l], never [r]. In final clusters composed of two members, the first consonant must be a nasal and the second a stop or fricative.

Relational Analysis

Comparison of AJ's productions with the adult target forms reveals only one error pattern that affects an entire class of sounds, i.e., constitutes a *phonological process*. The remaining errors affect specific sound segments and are described here as sound substitutions or deletions.

Phonological Process Error The only phonological process in AJ's sample is Vocalization, which affected both syllabic and nonsyllabic liquids in final position:

handle	ˈhændu	shower	ˈʃauwə
little	ˈlɪdu	zipper	ˈzɪpœ
nail	neu̯	jar	dʒaœ
spill	spɪu̯	chair	tʃɛœ

(In certain dialects of English, some of AJ's forms are an acceptable pronunciation. In the dialect AJ is acquiring, however, final /r/ and syllabic /r/ were produced with retroflexion.)

AJ also produced preconsonantal /l/ as a vowel; in contrast, preconsonantal /r/ as deleted, and the preceding vowel was lengthened:

/l/		/r/	
building	'bɪu̯dɪŋ	scared	skɛːd
milk	mɪu̯k	smart	smaːt
shelf	ʃɛu̯f	yard	jaːd

Sound Substitutions The sound substitutions in AJ's sample are described below.

1. **Adult /θ/ → Child [f]** The substitution of [f] for /θ/ occurs regularly in AJ's productions and is not affected by word position:

bathtub	'bæftʌb	think	fɪŋk
mouth	maʊf	three	fwi

2. **Adult /ð/ → Child [d]** The substitution of [d] for /ð/ occurred in productions of all words with target /ð/:

another	ə'nʌdə	them	dɛm
brother	'bwʌdə	this	dɪs

3. **Adult /ʃ/ → Child [s̩] in Medial and Final Position** Although AJ produces the palatal fricative /ʃ/ correctly in word-initial position, he substitutes a dental fricative [s̩] for this phoneme in other positions:

shelf	ʃɛu̯f	brush	bwʌs̩
shower	'ʃauwə	fish	fɪs̩

4. **Adult /r/ → Child [w] in Prevocalic Positions** The substitution of [w] for /r/ occurs frequently in AJ's words when /r/ is a singleton consonant and when it is part of a cluster. Some examples are:

brother	'bwʌdə	rush	wʌs̩
carry	'kɛwi	three	fwi

Optional Error Patterns Two additional patterns occur in AJ's sample—one involving deletion, the other insertion; both are optional (i.e., they do not occur in all possible cases). Final /r/, as shown above, was sometimes produced as a vowel, e.g., *chair* [tʃɛœ], and at other times it was deleted, e.g., *chair* [tʃɛ], *jar* [dʒa], *more* [mɔ]. The cluster /C + l/ was also produced variably, either correctly, e.g., *blood* [blʌd] and *flag* [flæg], or with [ə] inserted between the target consonants, e.g., *flag* [fəlæg], *play* [pəlei].

Comparison of Phonemic Systems

The adult phonemic contrasts for singleton consonants in word-initial and word-final position are compared with the contrasts in AJ's system in Figure 4.1. Differences between the two systems are indicated by circles in the display of AJ's phonemes.

When the two systems are displayed in this manner, called "item and replica" (Ferguson, 1968), it can be seen that the great majority of adult phonemic contrasts are rendered accurately in AJ's system. In word-initial position, there are just three exceptions: (1) adult /d/ and /ð/ are both produced as [d]; (2) adult /θ/ and /f/ are both [f]; and (3) adult /w/ and /r/ are both [w].

In final position, the difference between the two systems is not limited to mergers of target consonants; there are also several instances in which the phonemic contrast is maintained, but the phonetic realization of the contrastive units is not the same. The differences are: (1) adult /f/ and /θ/ are both produced [f], resulting in the loss of a contrast; (2) final /ʃ/ is produced [s̬], a phonetically distinct segment in AJ's productions that maintains the adult phonemic contrast even though the target consonant is not pronounced correctly; (3) final /r/ either is deleted, causing the loss of a contrast, or is produced as a vowel, in which case the contrast is maintained; and (4) final /l/ is produced as syllabic [u̬], a substitution that, although phonetically unlike the adult target, does maintain the target contrast.

The item-and-replica analysis (Figure 4.1) also indicates that certain phones in AJ's productions are in *complementary distribution* and should be regarded as allophones of a single phoneme. The palatal fricative [ʃ] occurs only word initially, whereas the dental fricative [s] occurs only word finally as a substitution for adult /ʃ/. Likewise /l/ occurs only in initial position and [u] only in final position (as a substitution for final /l/). In both cases the phones in AJ's productions should be regarded as allophones of one phoneme.

As in the case of SR, acoustic analyses of certain aspects of AJ's productions might reveal systematic differences between segments that were transcribed identically. For instance, the [w] of the words *rush* [wʌs̬] and *carry* [kɛwi] might differ from the [w] of *watch* or *wish*. Here again, as with SR, the corpus does not contain enough examples to make an acoustic analysis feasible. If one were desired, additional productions of specific contrasts would have to be elicited.

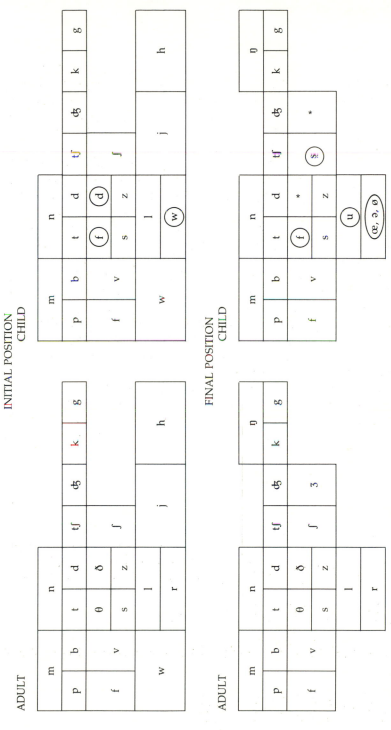

Figure 4.1 Contrastive phonemes using an item-and-replica model. Asterisk indicates the corpus included no adult words with this phoneme.

103

Summary

The analyses of SR's and AJ's speech samples illustrate various methods currently used in studying phonological development. The two basic types of analysis, independent and relational, provide a thorough picture of the two children's developing phonological systems. The independent analyses revealed the sounds and sound sequences produced. It was shown that SR's system was quite limited in terms of her inventory of phones, syllabic types, and possible sound sequences, whereas AJ's system was more fully developed and included a wide range of phones and syllabic types with few positional or sequential constraints.

The relational analyses revealed how closely the children's productions matched the adult model. In SR's sample the frequency of correct productions was relatively low due to the number of phonological processes ($n = 10$) and sound substitutions ($n = 2$) in her speech. The regular occurrence of the processes and substitutions resulted in the loss of many phonemic contrasts present in adult English. In contrast, a majority of AJ's pronunciations matched the adult model; few phonemic contrasts were lost, and only one phonological process was evident. The single-sound substitutions in his speech involved productions of liquids and fricatives, sound classes typically mastered relatively late.

In general, the analyses provided comprehensive descriptions of SR's and AJ's phonological system. However, there are some aspects of the descriptions that could be supplemented by acoustic analyses. As discussed, instrumental measurements of phonemic contrasts that were not maintained (according to the perceptual analysis) could reveal systematic distinctions between segments that were transcribed identically. If this were the case, a phonemic distinction would, in fact, be present even though it was imperceptible to the transcriber and probably to most other listeners as well.

Finally, the analyses for SR and AJ were limited to some extent by the nature of the sample. In both cases a continuous speech sample was used; as a result, some target phonemes were attempted only once or only in one position. In addition, the number and types of consonant clusters attempted was somewhat limited. As noted earlier, the only way to obtain a full range of target phonemes in all word positions is to use a predetermined word list for eliciting the speech sample. The disadvantages of word lists as the sole means of data collection were discussed earlier; however, in conjunction with a continuous speech sample, they can be used to elicit phonemes that otherwise might not occur.

Appendix:

Computer-Assisted Analyses

Not long ago computer-assisted phonological analyses were a dream of the future—now they are a reality. In addition to programs developed by researchers and clinicians for their personal use, there are now commercially available programs that can be used with small computers (e.g., Apple, IBM-PC) in clinical or university settings. Although relatively few programs are presently on the market, the number will undoubtedly increase dramatically in the near future, allowing users to select the one best designed for their specific needs. The purpose of this appendix is to examine the basic components of these programs and to discuss their use in clinical/research settings.

Input

Computerized programs differ in the amount of data that must be entered into the computer. If the sample to be analyzed is based on a predetermined list of words—usually a published articulation test—only the *child's pronunciation* of those words is entered. However, if analysis is based on a continuous speech sample, phonetic transcription of both the *adult model* and the *child's pronunciation* must be entered. In addition, an orthographic representation of each target word is usually included. Although it is possible to

105

note diacritical features, e.g., aspiration, nasalization, or rounding in the phonetic transcriptions (Stoel-Gammon, 1981; Stoel-Gammon et al., 1978), none of the programs currently available provides for this option.

Output

The computer is capable of carrying out major parts of the independent and relational analyses described in this chapter. Currently available programs can, for example, provide a complete inventory of phones produced by the child in various word positions. They can also compare the child's pronunciation with the adult model to: (1) determine instances of correct productions, omissions, and substitutions; (2) analyze substitution patterns in terms of a set of distinctive features; and (3) list the phonological processes used by the child and calculate the frequency of occurrence of each.

To our knowledge, none of the present programs provides an analysis of syllable structures or sequential constraints evident in the child's productions. In addition, analysis of substitution patterns and phonological processes are limited in some cases (see "Limitations," below).

Benefits

The primary advantage of computerized phonological analyses is that they save time. Once the phonetic transcriptions have been entered, the computer can carry out most (in some cases, all) of the desired analyses. Of course, the user (clinician/researcher) must still do the initial transcriptions, which can be time-consuming in its own right. In addition, because the programs are designed to compare the adult model and the child's pronunciation on a sound-by-sound basis, important decisions must be made when the transcribed data are typed into the computer. In essence, the user must determine the specific correspondences between the sounds of the child (see examples below).

The second advantage of using a computer is the accuracy with which it can perform needed arithmetic calculations. There is no doubt that a computer can count sounds and calculate percentages of occurrence more rapidly and more accurately than a person can.

Limitations

The major limitation of computerized phonological analyses is that the programs are designed to analyze the child's pronunciation of a target word by comparing it sound by sound with the adult model. Such comparisons allow the computer to identify instances of substitution and deletion and to determine occurrences of a set of phonological processes. In some cases, the sound-by-sound relationships between the two pronunciations are easy to determine; in others, there *is* no one-to-one correspondence between the sounds of the two forms. Consider, for example, the following productions:

Word	Child's form	Adult model (Child's form)
1. shoe	[su]	ʃu (su)
2. telephone	[dɛfõn]	t ɛləfon (dɛ fon)
3. spoon	[bũn]	spun (bun)
4. around	[wãʊ̃]	ər aʊnd (waʊ)
5. soup	[bup]	sup (bup)
6. bunny	[mʌni]	b ʌni (mʌni)
7. sweater	[dɛdə]	swɛr ɚ (d ɛdə)
8. swing	[fĩŋ]	swɪŋ (fɪŋ)
9. animal	[æmɪnl̩]	ænɪml̩ (æmɪnl̩)
10. basket	[bæksɪt]	bæskɪt (bæksɪt)

In the first four examples, the relationship between the sounds of the adult model and of the child's pronunciation seem to be relatively straightforward, and the substitution patterns and phonological processes are easily identified. (In example 4, however, some information present in the child's pronunciation is lost in the computerized analysis because the nasalization of the vowel, shown by a diacritic, is ignored by the computer.) The remaining examples (5–10) illustrate some of the problems of analyzing all productions on the basis of sound-by-sound correspondences.

In examples 5 (*soup* [bup]) and 6 (*bunny* [mʌni]), the initial consonants of the child's pronunciation can be analyzed in one of two ways—as simple substitutions ([b] for /s/ and [m] for /b/) or as instances of labial and nasal assimilation, respectively. Although the second alternative seems more likely, the decision should be based on an examination of other words in the speech sample to see if b/s or m/b occur as regular substitutions. Although a clinician or researcher can easily scan a sample to look for such substitutions, programming a computer to carry out this task is extremely difficult.

Examples 7 and 8 illustrate a different problem: When the child's pronunciation has one sound where the adult model has two, what is the relationship between the two forms? In many cases the correspondence seems clear, e.g., /s/ is deleted in [būn] for *spoon*, /r/ is deleted in [bɛd] for *bread*. In instances similar to those cited above, however, the sound correspondences are not so obvious. In the production of *sweater* as [dɛdə], it seems that the cluster /sw/ is reduced to a single consonant, which is then assimilated to the following [d]. However, does the initial sound of the child's form correspond to the /s/ or /w/ of the adult model? This decision must be made when the data are entered. In the child's production of the word *swing*, the initial cluster is treated differently in that the frication of /s/ is combined with the labiality of /w/ in a single segment [f] which is not a substitute for either the /s/ or /w/ of the adult form.

The final two examples, *animal* [æmɪnl] and *basket* [bæksɪt], are also problematic for the computer. Although they are actually instances of metathesis, the observed errors would be analyzed as straightforward substitutions (m/n–n/m and k/s–s/k) rather than as transpositions of target phonemes.

Summary

In sum, computer-assisted analyses can identify some (perhaps most) instances of speech-sound substitutions and omissions, but will incorrectly analyze some (perhaps most) occurrences of assimilation and metathesis. It is our view that the computer would provide a reliable analysis of children whose speech is characterized by relatively few errors or by common substitution patterns. At this time, however, it is not capable of adequately analyzing the productions of young, normally developing children (e.g., SR, whose speech sample was analyzed in this chapter) or children with severe phonological disorders (see DE and BC, who are discussed in Chapter 6). As the programs for phonological analysis become more sophisticated, they may be better able to handle productions that differ markedly from the target form; at present, however, they are limited in this domain.

Chapter 5

The Nature of Disordered Phonology

Although there are many conditions, e.g., mental retardation or hearing impairment, that have associated phonological problems, there is a population of children whose primary problem is phonological. These children are the primary focus of this chapter, although the concepts and techniques discussed can be applied to other children as well. The speech of phonologically disordered children is usually unintelligible and is characterized by many of the phonological processes described in Chapter 2. Identification of the etiology of the disorder is often difficult, although many possibilities have been offered. Suggested etiologies include: (1) auditory perceptual deficits (Van Riper, 1972; Winitz, 1975); (2) perceptual–motor deficits (McDonald, 1964; Shelton and Mc-Reynolds, 1979); or (3) linguistic deficits evident in abnormal sound patterns (Grunwell, 1981). Descriptions of children with phonological disorders are typically based on a single observation, often made at the time of the initial diagnosis of the disorder. Therefore, little is known about production during the prelinguistic or early linguistic periods of development, or about how the phonological system does or does not change over time.

Studies of phonologically disordered children have generally been of two types. In one type, the relationship between articulatory production and other variables (e.g., auditory discrimination skills, oral motor skills, personality, or reading skills) have been considered. These variables were primarily studied during the 1940s to 1960s. Some variables were consistently correlated with the occurrence of disordered phonology (e.g., auditory discrimination, oral motor skills for speech movements, and expressive language abilities), but no definitive etiology was identified. Bernthal and Bankson (1981) and Winitz (1969) provided comprehensive reviews of these studies. In the second type of study, the characteristics of segmental production are described primarily in terms of distinctive features and phonological rules (Compton, 1976; Crocker, 1969; Haas, 1963) or phonological processes (Dunn and Davis, 1983; Edwards and Bernhardt, 1973; Grunwell, 1981; Hodson and Paden, 1981).

The description of disordered phonology in this chapter focuses primarily on the second type of study, descriptions of segmental production. The characteristics of disordered phonology are described in two ways: (1) productions are examined as a self-contained system (the *independent analysis* described in Chapter 4); and (2) they are compared with the adult model (*relational analysis*). Other characteristics related to speech production are also described. Finally, the phonology of disordered children is compared with that of normal children.

Independent Analysis

Phonetic Inventory

The phonetic inventory is a list of phones produced without reference to whether or not they are used correctly. An inventory of phones produced by disordered children (ages 2;7–8;0) has been described in three studies (Grunwell, 1981; Ingram, 1981; Schwartz et al., 1980). When the inventories for all 25 children were compared, the results were remarkably similar. The following phones occurred in over half of the samples:

Stops	p	b	t	d	k	g	
Fricatives	f		s				
Nasals		m		n			
Glides		w					h

Stops, nasals, and fricatives were the most frequently produced manner features; labial, alveolar, and velar were the most frequent place features. The phones were produced more frequently in initial than in medial or final positions for all children.

The inventory above can be compared to the ones presented in Chapter 2 for the three normal children Daniel, Sarah, and Will, who were between the ages of 11 and 17 months. The inventories are similar in the number of sounds included (10 for the normal children and 12 for the disordered children). They are also similar in the sounds that first occurred consistently (i.e., stops, nasals, glides, and a few fricatives). Both groups produced sounds across a variety of sound classes. In these ways, the inventory of the disordered children is similar to those of the normal children.

However, the inventory above does not fully represent the range of phones that occurred. A majority of children produced other English and non-English phones, but they did not occur in enough samples to be included in the inventory above. Therefore, although there was a group of phones that characterized the children's consonant repertoire, there were differences among the individual children. Most children had very limited inventories (about half the number of possible English phones), but there was a tendency for older children to have more phones in the inventory.

Syllable and Word Shape

When considering the syllable shapes of words, CV (consonant–vowel) and CVC were the shapes produced most frequently by 20 disordered children studied by Grunwell (1981), Schwartz et al. (1980), and Shriberg and Kwiatkowski (1980). These shapes were used in both mono- and multisyllabic words. They are shapes similar to those used by the three normal children described in Chapter 2 who were in the single-word stage. Grunwell (1981) reported that sequences of consonants, such as clusters (e.g., CCV, VCC) or abutting consonants within a word (e.g., CVCCV), are rarely produced by unintelligible children. She pointed out that her data showed "how different the child's usage of syllable structure is from the normal adult usage." As the unintelligible children develop larger productive lexicons that include multisyllabic words, the syllable structure fails to become more complex. However, children who are more intelligible do produce some consonant clusters (Dunn and Davis, 1983) and abutting consonants (Dunn, 1983).

Relational Analysis

Phonological Processes

A variety of analyses have been used to describe the relationship between the disordered child's productions and the adult form. The analyses have been based on single sounds, phonological rules written in distinctive features, and phonological processes. The latter have been adopted as our framework for describing error patterns because they provide more comprehensive descriptions than other approaches. As mentioned in Chapter 2, phonological processes provide a means for describing, but not explaining, the error patterns evident in young children's speech.

In order to describe and compare error patterns in phonologically disordered children, eight studies were selected for review (Compton, 1976; Dunn and Davis, 1983; Edwards and Bernhardt, 1973; Grunwell, 1981; Hodson and Paden, 1981; McReynolds and Elbert, 1981; Schwartz et al., 1980; Shriberg and Kwiatkowski, 1980). These studies provide results from more than 120 children with multiple errors, ranging in age from 2;8 to 13 years. There were differences across these studies in subject selection criteria (age, severity, amount of time in treatment), data collection procedures (single word versus conversational sampling), and analytical procedures (phonological rule versus process description; inclusion and definition of different error patterns). Despite these differences, it was possible to identify commonalities in occurrence of phonological processes. The majority of studies reported *which* processes occurred for each child but not *how frequently*. Therefore Table 5.1 presents percentages of occurrence based on the number of children who demonstrated the process. Although many processes were described in the studies, only those that occurred in five or more of the studies are included.

Nine processes occurred most frequently among these children. The first three processes in Table 5.1—Cluster Reduction, Final Consonant Deletion, and Unstressed Syllable Deletion—are processes that modify the syllable structure of the target word. The next four processes—Stopping, Velar and Palatal Fronting, and Liquid Simplification—are substitution processes. Palatal Fronting is the substitution of a front consonant (e.g., alveolar, labial) for palatal fricatives and affricates. Liquid Simplification is the combination of the processes Gliding and Vocalization. The last two processes, Assimilation and Voicing, involve sound changes

Table 5.1 Percentage of Children in Each Study Who Demonstrated the Phonological Process

Process	Compton (1976) (n = 20) 5;0–6;0	Edwards & Bernhardt (1973) (n = 4) 3;3–5;3	Dunn & Davis (1983) (n = 9) 3;8–5;10	Grunwell (1981) (n = 7) 5;0–8;0	Hodson & Paden (1981) (n = 60) 3;0–8;0	McReynolds & Elbert (1981) (n = 13) 3;7–13;0	Schwartz et al. (1980) (n = 3) 2;7–3;7	Shriberg & Kwiatkowski (1980) (n = 12) 4;0–7;6
Cluster Reduction (CR)	100	100	100	100	100	100	100	100
Final Consonant Deletion (FCD)	75	50	100	86	50	100	100	83
Unstressed Syllable Deletion (USD)	—[a]	25	100	100	67	54	67	67
Stopping (S)	100	100	100	86	100	77	100	91
Velar Fronting (VF)	40	50	100	71	67	67	100	33
Palatal Fronting (PF)	75	100	—[b]	71	—[a]	—[b]	—[b]	16
Liquid Simplification (LS)[c]	95	100	100	86	100	100	67	50
Assimilation (ASS)	—[a]	100	44	71	100	54	100	58
Voicing Processes (Vc)	40-I 65-F	100	—[a]	57	67-I	92	100	—[a]

[a] No data available.

[b] Velar and palatal fronting combined.

[c] A combination of Gliding and Vocalization.

in which one sound becomes more like another. In Table 5.1 Assimilation is a combination of all types (e.g., labial, nasal, velar).

There were variations in results across the studies, but general trends can be observed. Cluster Reduction occurred in all children, suggesting that regardless of differences in age, sampling techniques, or type of analysis phonologically disordered children had difficulty producing consonant clusters. Stopping and Liquid Simplification occurred with high levels of frequency across children, indicating that these children also had difficulty producing fricatives and liquids. Assimilation and Voicing changes occurred with the next greatest frequency. The four remaining processes, Final Consonant Deletion, Unstressed Syllable Deletion, and Velar and Palatal Fronting, varied more in frequency of occurrence than the other processes. It is possible that these four processes never occurred in some of the children's speech or had been eliminated.

The patterns of occurrence of processes in disordered children are very similar to those described in Chapter 2 for normal children. The processes that tended to be most widespread and persistently used by the two groups are similar (Cluster Reduction, Liquid Simplification, and Stopping). Other processes tended to vary in occurrence across both groups of children, particularly Assimilation and Velar Fronting.

Although the data in Table 5.1 illustrate the major trends in frequency of occurrence of phonological processes, they do not address other important issues. First, many other processes were reported to occur in the speech of these children. Thus although a few processes may characterize a majority of the error patterns of disordered children, there is great variability in the range of processes that occur. Another issue concerns how frequently an error must occur in a speech sample or how many sounds in a sound class must be affected before the error is labeled a process. No criteria have been established for these issues, so the results of each study differ. Finally, there is little information about how frequently a process occurs for individual children. This is important because many children may have a process (e.g., Assimilation) but it may occur only three or four times in the child's speech. Thus the process would have little significance in the child's system.

Dunn and Davis (1983) studied the occurrence of phonological processes in the continuous speech of 9 disordered children, ages 3;8–5;10. There were seven processes (Table 5.2) that occurred most frequently; in fact, they accounted for 65% of all errors. The percentage of occurrence of each process for individual children was derived by dividing the number of actual occurrences by the

Table 5.2 Percentage of Occurrences for Each Phonological Process for Individual Subjects

Subject	ASS[a]	Red[a]	USD	S	FCD	VF	Dep	LS	CR
1	0	0	9	25	23	73	55	79	68
2	2	0	21	21	35	3	15	83	47
3	1	0	8	61	60	54	0	92	100
4	1	0	22	20	52	0	0	7	53
5	0	0	19	12	21	67	17	71	68
6	0	0	12	20	11	11	50	90	79
7	0	1	2	12	45	68	64	70	86
8	0	0	8	15	35	16	15	78	65
9	1	0	7	3	34	3	82	32	84

Adapted from Dunn and Davis (1983). See Table 5.1 for explanations of abbreviations.

[a]Potential occurrences and percentages were not identified for assimilation (Ass) or reduplication (Red) because by definition these processes could occur several times per word. The numbers for these processes are actual occurrences.

number of potential occurrences. Even though seven of the processes occurred in all of the samples, there was a great deal of individual variation across children. For example, Liquid Simplification occurred in 92% of the possible target words for subject 3 but in only 7% of the possible words for subject 4 (Table 5.2). Another aspect of these results is the low percentage of occurrence of some processes. For example, if the Stopping score of subject 3 (the subject with the most unintelligible speech) is omitted, the percentage of occurrence for the group ranged from 3 to 25%. Even though Stopping occurred in all samples, it was not particularly significant in the system of any child except subject 3. The results of this study illustrate the importance of reporting the frequency of occurrence of each process for individual children; without this information, children's errors cannot be adequately interpreted. Finally, the results show once again that, although a few common phonological processes occur in the samples of most children, there is great variation in the occurrence of most processes.

Idiosyncratic Processes

Another group of processes, referred to as *idiosyncratic*, has been identified in the speech of phonologically disordered children. Idiosyncratic processes have been described as those error patterns that have never been documented in normal children or that occur

Table 5.3 Idiosyncratic Processes that Occur in the Speech of Phonologically Disordered Children

Process	Description
Atypical Cluster Reduction	Deletion of the member that is usually retained: [ren] for *train;* [sap] for *stop*
Initial Consonant Deletion	Deletion of a singleton consonant in the initial position of a word: [ep] for *tape*
Glottal Replacement	Substitution of a glottal stop for a consonant, usually in medial or final position: [læ?ɚ] for *ladder*
Backing	Substitution of a velar consonant for a more anterior consonant: [pæk] for *pat*
Fricatives substituted for stops	Substitution of a fricative consonant for a stop consonant: [sændḷ] for *candle*
Stops substituted for glides	Substitution of a stop consonant for a glide consonant [bɪl] for *will*
Sound Preference	Substitution of one consonant for several other consonants, in an unpredictable pattern: substitution of [f] for most initial fricatives and affricates and for initial stops in /stop + r/ clusters

infrequently in the normal population. Examples of the more frequently identified idiosyncratic processes are provided in Table 5.3, based on studies of Dunn and Davis (1983), Edwards and Bernhardt (1973), Grunwell (1981), Ingram (1976), and Weiner (1981a). The first two processes in the table are syllable structure processes. Atypical Cluster Reduction refers to the deletion of the member that is *usually* maintained by children (e.g., deletion of the stop rather than the liquid, in a /stop + liquid/ cluster). The remaining processes are substitution processes: Glottal Replacement, Backing, Fricatives substituted for stops, Stops substituted for glides, and Sound Preference. Sound Preference is the substitution of one consonant for several other consonants. For example, Weiner (1981a) described a child who substituted [h] for initial voiceless fricatives and stops whether the consonants occurred as singletons or in clusters (e.g., [haɪv] for *five;* ['hebo] for *table*). Another example is the substitution of [f] for most initial fricatives and affricates and for initial stops in /stop + r/ clusters, e.g., ['fibʊ] for *zebra* and ['frʌ?ɪ?] for *brushing* (Edwards, 1980b). The occurrence of Sound Preference significantly alters intelligibility because it neutralizes contrasts in the child's speech.

The variety and frequency of occurrence of idiosyncratic processes in phonologically disordered children have not been systematically documented. It seems that most disordered children have at least one or two such processes in addition to the nine processes reviewed earlier (Table 5.1). The presence of idiosyncratic processes may indicate that the disorder is more severe. At the same time, these processes may indicate creative strategies that children use to master the phonological system. Further study will indicate whether the idiosyncratic processes have prognostic value and if they are more difficult than "normal" processes to eliminate.

Vowel Production

In descriptions of disordered phonology, vowels are rarely mentioned as part of the problem. This lack of attention to vowels leaves the impression that vowels are rarely in error. When vowels are misarticulated, they are usually viewed as part of a larger phonological or language problem, and the vowel errors are not described in any detail (Grunwell, 1981; Ingram, 1976; Renfrew, 1966). In a case study that described a child who misarticulated vowels, Hargrove (1982) observed that practicing speech-language pathologists describe vowel errors as being more common than indicated in the literature. She encouraged the study of vowels in the speech of disordered children in order to determine "whether the perception that vowel misarticulations are rare is due to (a) a low incidence or (b) a general insensitivity on the part of speech-language pathologists to vowel misarticulations."

Phonemic Contrasts

A major goal of phonological acquisition is the use of sounds to contrast meaning. For example, in the words *fan* and *pan*, the phonemes /f/ and /p/ are contrastive. Although little has been written about contrastive ability in phonologically disordered children, Grunwell (1980) described poor contrastive ability as one of the major characteristics of disordered phonology. One reason for lack of contrast may be a small phonetic inventory; if there are few phones in a child's productive repertoire, the potential for contrast is limited. In addition to lack of potential for contrast, Grunwell (1980) observed that disordered children often fail to use the potential they have. That is, they do not use the sounds they can produce in a contrastive way. For example, a child may be able to *produce* /f/ but substitutes [p] for /f/ in initial word position, failing to maintain a potential contrast.

It is important to understand the reasons for the failure to maintain contrasts. In the case of a small phonetic inventory, the reason for lack of contrasts may be difficulty with the production of sounds. In the case of failure to use sounds contrastively, children may lack knowledge about the contrastive function of phones or may not have categorized two consonants as separate phonemes. In the latter case, phones would probably occur in free variation, e.g., [f] alternating with [p].

Disordered children may know that two phonemes are contrastive and yet may not be able to *produce* the sounds. To solve this problem, children may develop unorthodox ways of maintaining the contrast. For example, a child may be unable to produce final voiced obstruent consonants. In order to maintain a contrast among words ending in these consonants, the child may prolong the vowel that would occur before the voiced consonant, e.g., *bag*–[bæ:k] versus *back*–[bæk]. This vowel-lengthening is similar to that used by normal children, as described in Chapter 2. In other instances, a child may have contrasts that are not perceptible to the listener; that is, there may be subtle differences in production that would be apparent only with instrumental analysis. Maxwell and Weismer (1982) described a child, age 3;11, who substituted [d] for 20 different sounds or sound sequences, e.g., /s, g, kr, tw/. Spectrographic analysis revealed that the productions of words with these 20 adult sounds could be grouped into three categories based on three significantly different voice onset times: (1) words beginning with an adult /d/ (*dog*); (2) words beginning with voiced obstruents other than /d/ (*zoo, grew*); and (3) words beginning with voiceless obstruents (*too, crew*). These results provide an example of a child who apparently had knowledge of differences in voicing characteristics of consonants but could not produce those differences in an adult-like way. He developed an unusual way to maintain differences that were not perceptible to the adult listener.

Variability in Production

Variability is another factor that contributes to understanding the nature of disordered phonology. Disordered children are often characterized as highly variable in production of phonemes and words (Grunwell, 1981; Edwards and Bernhardt, 1973; Lorentz, 1974, 1976). The framework below represents the types of variability that have been described in the literature.

1. Variability in the production of a phone *across* different lexical items:

[s]	sun	tʌn
	soap	ʃop
	suit	sut
	sit	dɪt

2. Variability in the production of a phone *within* the same lexical item:

[s]	sun	sʌn
		tʌn
		dʌn

3. Variability in the production of several sounds across several words (a combination of types 1 and 2):

sun	sʌn	shoe	su	chick	sɪk
	tʌn		tu		tɪk
	dʌn		du		dɪk
	ʃʌn		ʃu		ʃɪk

Grunwell (1981) referred to the third example as "almost complete unpredictability."

Descriptions of variability in disordered phonology have differed, and at first glance the descriptions seem contradictory. For example, Grunwell (1981) reported that the seven children she studied were extremely variable. The variability was primarily type 1 above (across words), rather than type 2 or 3. Lorentz (1974) described one child as having variation in the production of almost every phoneme in the sample. This widespread variability was possibly type 3. In contrast to these two examples, Lorentz stated elsewhere (1976) that "aberrant phonological systems of four- and five-year-old children are relatively fixed and consistent." He went on to say that when a disordered system begins to change there is an increase in variability and incorrect production. It is possible that these three descriptions represent a continuum of variability: (1) little or no variability; (2) variability without improved accuracy; (3) variability that includes correct production; and (4) correct production. Children may progress through this continuum or may plateau at any point and not progress toward consistently correct use of a phone. This continuum is offered as a possible explanation for the discrepant descriptions that have appeared in the literature on disordered phonology. Although there is little systematic evidence to support the continuum, such information is potentially very useful. Different types of variability may be identified and used to predict success in remediation.

There are many factors that can influence the types of variability described above: several of these were mentioned in Chapter 4. Those factors included: (1) type of elicitation procedure used (e.g., imitation versus spontaneous production); (2) production of a sound in a single word or in continuous speech, where the phonetic context may influence correct production; (3) word length; (4) familiarity with a word; and (5) the status of a sound in the course of acquisition (sounds progressing toward mastery may be more variable). An additional factor is linguistic complexity; as utterances become longer and more complex syntactically, children often reduce words phonologically (Panagos et al., 1979).

Comparison of Normal and Disordered Children

Direct comparisons of the phonological characteristics of normal and disordered children have been made by Ingram (1980) and Schwartz et al. (1980). The normal children in both studies were 17–26 months of age, whereas the disordered children were 3–8 years. In the Ingram study the normal and disordered children were matched by their Articulation Scores, which is a weighted score based on the number of sounds in the phonetic inventory. The children in the Schwartz et al. study were matched for sex and mean length of utterance. No information was provided about the language skills of Ingram's disordered group; those in the Schwartz et al. group were at least 15 months below age level on the language portion of the Lexington Developmental Scale. In each study the normal and disordered children were highly similar in the most frequent types of sounds that occurred in their phonetic inventories and syllable shapes that were produced. The Schwartz et al. results also revealed that the phonological processes demonstrated by the two groups were very similar. When these authors considered variability in productions, they observed no differences in frequency of optional processes or in the variation of productions within words. Schwartz et al. concluded that differences are not found when data from disordered children are compared with data from normal children at similar early levels in linguistic development. The results of these two studies indicate that the phonological characteristics of some disordered children are similar to 18- to 24-month-old children developing language normally.

Hodson and Paden (1981) obtained somewhat different but not contradictory results when they compared the occurrence of phonological processes in two groups of children. One group was normally developing (age 4–5 years), whereas the other group was unintelligible and thus severely disordered (age 3–8 years). The disordered children had frequent occurrence of processes demonstrated by young normal children, e.g., Cluster Reduction, Stopping, and Velar Fronting. The normal children demonstrated none of these processes; instead, they primarily had single-sound errors, e.g., substitutions for /θ, ð, l, ɝ/. Obviously, the phonological characteristics of the disordered children were no longer similar to those of normal children. These three comparison studies show that disordered children may begin with phonological characteristics that are very similar to those of normal children, but, at some point in the process of acquisition, development is arrested or begins to follow a course different from that of normal acquisition.

Many other people have attempted to characterize the relationship between normal and disordered phonology on the basis of clinical and research evidence (Compton, 1976; Edwards and Bernhardt, 1973; Grunwell, 1981; Ingram, 1976; Leonard, 1973; Oller, 1973). These authors concurred that the phonological characteristics (e.g., sounds, rules, processes) of normal and disordered children are similar but that there are also substantial differences. The most frequently described differences in disordered phonology include:

1. Static systems that plateau at an early level of development, failing to progress toward mastery.
2. Extreme variability in production, without gradual improvement in production.
3. Persistence of phonological processes beyond the expected ages of occurrence in normal children.
4. Co-occurrence of processes that are observed early in normal acquisition (e.g., Reduplication or Final Consonant Deletion) with correct production of sounds that are normally acquired late in the sequence of acquisition (e.g., liquids, fricatives, clusters); Grunwell (1981) referred to this pattern as *Chronological Mismatch*.
5. Occurrence of idiosyncratic rules or processes, which rarely occur in normal phonology; these processes significantly reduce intelligibility.
6. Restricted use of contrast.

The majority of these differences has been derived from a few case studies. It is not clear if all disordered children have all of these characteristics or if there are subgroups of children who demonstrate selected characteristics.

The possibility that there are some children who may not exhibit all of these characteristics raises the issue of *deviance* versus *delay*. Some authors (Ingram, 1976; Leonard, 1973) have suggested that phonologically disordered children can be divided into two groups, a delayed group and a deviant group. One implication is that the delayed group does not need treatment, whereas the deviant group does. The problem with these categories is that they are poorly defined and have not been empirically supported (Grunwell, 1981). For example, Ingram (1976) referred to "deviant children" as those "who require therapy" because they "acquire a phonological system in a unique way, showing patterns of acquisition that never appear in young normal children." It is not clear what these unique patterns are, so it is difficult to project a priori whether a child needs treatment. In addition, there are not enough data from normal children to unequivocally determine that certain patterns never occur during normal acquisition. In fact, many of the processes labeled as "idiosyncratic" in Table 5.3 have been reported as occurring in the speech of normally developing children. It is possible that disordered children differ from normal children in the *way* that the patterns are used (e.g., the patterns persist, or lack contrastive function). In other words, the difference between normal and disordered children may be in the *process* of acquisition rather than in the *product* (i.e., phones produced or processes used). At this time, identification of deviant versus delayed children is difficult because of a lack of firm criteria for assignment to either group.

Related Skills in Children with Disordered Phonology

There are variables that relate to the etiology of disordered phonology and that may be the underlying reasons for the characteristic patterns of production in disordered children. Variables to be discussed include: (1) speech perception; (2) oral motor skills; and (3) language skills.

Speech Perception

Speech perception is typically measured by having disordered children discriminate between phones presented in word or nonsense-syllable pairs that differ in one phoneme (e.g., *wing–ring*). Results of studies that evaluated discrimination abilities are equivocal (Winitz, 1969), suggesting that some, but not all, disordered children have difficulty with speech discrimination. Instead of a global discrimination problem, difficulty may lie in discriminating *error* sounds from other sounds. Some children may fail to differentiate their error productions from target productions (Locke, 1980a,b) but this difficulty is not universal (McReynolds et al., 1975).

Other auditory skills have been tested in addition to discrimination testing, e.g., short-term memory or auditory sequencing. Phonologically disordered children as a group have not had difficulty with these skills. Therefore, given all the results of testing speech perception skills, some authors have concluded that auditory deficits are not a characteristic of phonologically disordered children (Grunwell, 1980). However, a word of caution must be added. First, some errors in phonemic perception may occur as late as age 8 in normal children (Templin, 1957); therefore the same acquisition patterns would occur in disordered children as well. In addition, testing techniques are often gross and thus possibly fail to identify subtle auditory deficits. When more refined measurement procedures are used, underlying auditory knowledge may be revealed. For example, in the Maxwell and Weismer (1982) study reviewed earlier, spectrographic analysis revealed underlying knowledge of distinctions among sounds. The child was apparently able to differentiate auditorily among sounds that he could not produce.

Nature of Underlying Representation The discussion of perceptual ability is related to a broader issue about disordered children's phonological knowledge. This issue involves the way in which children internally store words, referred to in Chapter 3 as the *underlying representation*. Most descriptions of disordered phonology do not address this issue and thus imply that children's underlying representations are the same as the adult spoken form. In other words, it is assumed that children perceive and store words correctly. Recently, however, empirical evidence has indicated that children's underlying representations may not always be the adult form. Macken (1980b) cited evidence that some errors can be explained only by misperception and suggested that in such cases underlying representation is different from the adult form. As mentioned in Chapter 3, Dinnsen et al. (1979) analyzed production errors in an attempt to determine the nature of the "productive" underlying representation.

Information about productive and perceptual abilities is important because one cannot directly test a child's underlying knowledge. Children with adult-like underlying representations probably do not need to be taught perceptual skills; instead they apparently need articulatory practice. On the other hand, children whose underlying representations do not match adult forms will need to learn accurate representation of those adult forms, either from auditory perceptual or phonemic contrast training. In sum, description of the underlying representations of phonologically disordered children is an important aspect of characterizing the disorder.

Oral Motor Skills

Deficits in oral motor skills have been proposed as an underlying cause of disordered phonology (McDonald, 1964). Empirical evidence that identifies the nature of the oral motor deficit is lacking. Phonologically disordered children often perform more poorly than normal children on nonspeech and speech tasks. For example, disordered children repeated combinations of nonsense syllables more slowly than normal children (McNutt, 1977). However, normal children are successful speakers, whereas disordered children have histories of failure with speech; this history places them at a disadvantage in a task that requires maximal production in a timed situation. The relationship between the ability to produce repeated sequences of nonsense syllables (referred to as diadochokinesis) and production in conversational speech is unclear, because the movements required in these two tasks are so different (McDonald, 1964).

There are certainly children who have oral motor involvement. For example, even when given a model to imitate and cues about how to produce a target sound, some children are not successful. This difficulty is indicative of some kind of motoric immaturity or deficit. These children should be differentiated from children who can *produce* the sounds but fail to use the sounds to maintain contrasts.

Language Skills

The language skills of phonologically disordered children have been measured to determine if language and phonological disorders co-exist. The language skills that have been studied ranged from general abilities (e.g., mean length of utterance, comprehension of sentences) to specific skills (e.g., use of selected syntactic structures). Aram and Kamhi (1982) provided a thorough review of studies that relate phonology and language. Conclusive results have not emerged from the studies, in large part because of differences in subject selection criteria and the language measures used.

In general, phonological and language disorders coexist in many children but not in all. The results consistently revealed that: (1) comprehension of linguistic structures was not often affected (Shriberg, 1982b); and (2) syntactic deficits co-occurred with phonological problems more frequently than deficits in other linguistic skills. Some children possibly have difficulty mastering *expressive linguistic form*, which might include the form of reading and writing, as well as phonology, morphology, and syntax (Dunn et al., 1983). Aram and Kamhi (1982) concluded that there is not yet a clear understanding about the relationship between co-occurrence of phonological and language disorders. They discussed three possible explanations for the co-occurrence: (1) linguistic (e.g., difficulty in forming linguistic categories and rules); (2) cognitive (e.g., difficulty in hypothesis testing and problem-solving abilities); or (3) information processing (e.g., difficulty with processing, e.g., discrimination, storage, or retrieval of linguistic information). Longitudinal case studies would provide information about the co-occurrence of phonological and language deficits, and possible explanations for their co-occurrence.

Summary

A variety of potential deficits has been mentioned in the literature as possible explanations for phonological disorders. The deficit areas include speech perception, oral motor skills, and linguistic abilities. There is a lack of evidence that clearly implicates any one of these areas in all disordered children. Instead, the results of many empirical studies indicate that deficiencies in any or all of these skills may coexist with disordered phonology, but the coexistence of skills or deficits does not explain the cause of phonological disorders. A great deal of research is needed to identify the specific nature of variables that co-occur with and influence phonological disorders.

Conclusions

In many respects, children with severe phonological disorders have similar speech characteristics. They typically have a reduced inventory of sounds, and the syllable structure of their words is simple. Like normal children, disordered children are least accurate in their production of fricatives, affricates, liquids, and clusters. A large proportion of their errors can be described in terms of a limited number of phonological processes. The processes are similar to those observed in normal children. Disordered children also have persistent idiosyncratic processes that occur infrequently for brief periods in normal children. In addition, some disordered children may have a different sequence of acquisition from normal children in that they correctly produce one or more later-developing phonemes while failing to produce some earlier-developing ones. Finally, disordered children often fail to maintain phonemic contrasts, either because they have a small inventory or because they have a large inventory but use it incorrectly.

The nature of disordered phonology may be most accurately characterized by the manner in which these children proceed through the acquisition process. Such children have been described as highly variable in their productions. However, the variability often does not seem to lead to mastery, as it often does in normal children because variability does not give way to correct production. In many cases, phonologically disordered children seem to have plateaued in acquisition because they persist in using immature patterns and/or form idiosyncratic ways of coping with word production. These children may have other etiological deficits that are related to the phonological deficit, including problems with speech perception, oral motor skills, and expressive language. In addition, deficits with abilities such as storage, retrieval, organization, and sequencing of phonological (or linguistic) symbols may also contribute to the etiology of disordered phonology.

There is an additional point that should be made about the characteristics of disordered phonology. Although phonologically disordered children have been described as being similar, in fact they are also very different from one another. For example, disordered children often have similar phonetic inventories, but the sounds emerge in different word positions and are mastered at different times. In addition, these children tend to differ in the idiosyncratic patterns that occur in their speech. In sum, no two disordered children present precisely the same patterns nor will they proceed through the stages of phonological acquisition in exactly the same way. It is necessary to identify the unique characteristics of each child's system in order to design the most appropriate treatment plan for each child.

Chapter 6

Assessment of Disordered Phonology

Assessment of phonology in children has four basic objectives. These objectives are hierarchically related, so that one must be completed in order to provide sufficient information for the next objective to be realized. The first objective is to determine if there is a phonological disorder. If a disorder is diagnosed, the next objective is to make recommendations for management, e.g., referral to another professional or enrollment in treatment. If treatment is recommended, the next objective is to make suggestions for specific treatment goals. The final objective is to assess the child's progress during treatment. The first three objectives provide the basis for this chapter, and the last is discussed in Chapter 7.

The first and primary objective of assessment—formulation of a diagnosis—culminates in a decision about whether there is a problem and its possible etiology. In order to make this decision, it is necessary to: (1) collect a speech sample; (2) analyze the sample; and (3) integrate the analyses with other testing results and normative data. Each of these steps is discussed in this chapter; two case studies are presented to illustrate the implementation of each step and the formulation of a diagnostic statement. The analyses for the cases are used as a basis for discussing the second and third objectives: recommendations for management of the problem and selection of treatment goals.

Model for Phonological Assessment

When conducting a phonological assessment, it is important that phonology be considered in a broad framework of other skills. This can be done by developing a model that includes reference to the skills that a child must have to perceive and produce the patterns of adult phonology. This model should serve as the guiding framework for assessment and diagnosis, so that, ideally, all factors that contribute to the phonological disorder will be identified. If a variety of factors are not considered, their influence on phonological skills cannot be identified and treatment cannot include information essential to improvement. For example, a phonological disorder may be part of a broader problem, e.g., a language disorder.

As discussed in Chapter 3, there is no model that adequately describes all abilities necessary for phonological acquisition. However, we have proposed some basic components that should be included in a model: (1) auditory perceptual; (2) cognitive; (3) phonological; and (4) neuromotor. The assessment of these abilities is discussed as part of supplementary testing and is integrated with the results of phonological assessment for each case study.

Collection of a Sample

The first step in forming a diagnostic statement is the collection of a sample. There are three common ways of obtaining a sample from phonologically disordered children: single-word articulation tests, sentence articulation tests, and continuous speech samples. These sampling procedures were discussed in Chapter 3, except for sentence tests; their use with disordered children is presented below.

Single-Word Tests

In single-word sampling, a set of words is elicited that contains all consonants of English in initial, medial, and final word positions. Phonemes are evaluated as both single sounds and clusters; vowels are sometimes assessed as well. Test stimuli are usually pictures of nouns. The results of a single-word test provide information about production of sounds and the child's ability to match adult forms. Additional uses for single-word articulation tests include:

1. Rapid measurement of the child's ability to produce all the sounds of English.
2. Comparison of results with normative data (e.g., Sander, 1972; Templin, 1957) to determine if the child is within normal limits for production of sounds in single words.
3. For the unintelligible child, production of a predetermined set of words is necessary in order to have an identifiable sample for describing the child's phonological system.
4. Readministration of the test to measure progress after a period of treatment.
5. Comparison of single-word productions with production of words from a continuous speech sample.

In the design of articulation tests, it is important to consider the effect of linguistic characteristics (e.g., grammatical role and morphophonemic factors) and canonical shapes of words tested. These factors can influence the accuracy of production (Shriberg and Kwiatkowski, 1980). Another factor to consider in word selection is the effect that one part of a word might have on another. For example, the occurrence of a velar in a word might result in Velar Assimilation; thus the /tʃ/ in *chicken* would be produced as [k]: ['kɪkən]. In words without the velar influence, the /tʃ/ might be correct or have another more typical substitution. Currently, only one single-word test, the Assessment of Phonological Processes (Hodson, 1980), provides for analysis of the influence of the canonical shape and the relationship of consonants in a word, as well as other systematic substitution and deletion patterns.

In the Hodson procedure, objects are used to elicit production of 55 words. The test results are organized according to: (1) basic phonological processes (Syllable Reduction, Cluster Reduction, Singleton Obstruent Omission, Stridency Deletion, Velar Deviations); (2) miscellaneous phonological processes (Glottal Replacement, Stopping, etc., for a total of 12 processes in this category); (3) Sonorant Deviations; (4) Assimilation processes; and (5) articulatory shifts (single-sound substitutions and distortions). There are multiple opportunities for the majority of the processes to occur, making it possible to obtain a percentage of occurrence for most processes. Hodson's assessment procedure is intended for unintelligible children who have multiple errors that can be described as processes.

There are other limitations of a single-word sampling procedure. Some of these were discussed in Chapter 4; the major reservations pertaining to disordered children are:

1. Limited number of productions per phoneme (e.g., once in word initial, medial and final positions) fail to reveal information about variability.
2. Patterns that are representative of a child's abilities may fail to occur, whereas atypical errors may be "triggered" owing to the words on the test (Shriberg and Kwiatkowski, 1980).
3. Both spontaneous and imitative responses are often obtained, making interpretation of results difficult.
4. Single-word productions are not affected by words in the surrounding context, so they are often less representative of typical speech patterns than words in continuous speech (Faircloth and Faircloth, 1970).

These limitations are great enough that a single-word test cannot accurately reflect the child's phonological ability. An articulation test can be a useful supplement to the analysis of a continuous sample. For example, comparison of productions in the two conditions can provide information about the severity of the disorder. The child who has fewer sounds in error on the test than in the continuous sample is less severely involved than the child who has the same errors in both conditions.

Sentence Articulation Tests

In sentence articulation tests, single consonants, consonant clusters, and vowels are elicited by having the person read sentences. These tests are appropriate for persons with a reading level specified by the test, typically second or third grade level. Sentence tests have many of the same limitations that single-word tests have, except that they do allow for production of sounds in continuous speaking contexts. The sounds are produced spontaneously on a sentence test, but the effect of the written form in cueing a correct response is not known. A limitation of many of these tests is that the sentences are "loaded" with the same or similar sounds; this technique results in very complex sound sequences. For example, the following sentence from The Fisher-Logemann Test of Articulation Competence (Fisher and Logemann, 1971) tests /s/ and /z/: "Suzie sewed zippers on two new dresses at Bessie's house." Production of such sentences may result in atypical errors. However, sentence tests are useful for quickly identifying specific errors and are valuable when administered in conjunction with collection of a continuous speech sample.

Continuous Speech Sample

Our preference for sampling the phonology of disordered children is the collection of a continuous speech sample. This sample is typically collected in a clinical or school setting, using familiar objects to elicit continuous speech. The objects used to collect the sample can represent words selected to include: (1) a variety of canonical shapes; (2) consonants that occur infrequently in samples, e.g., fricatives and affricates; and (3) consonants that are particularly desired for analysis. It is preferable to have 80–100 words for analysis (Ingram, 1981; Shriberg and Kwiatkowski, 1980). The number of utterances required to elicit 100 different words varies according to the child's lexicon, mean length of utterance, and willingness to talk during the sample. Fifty utterances are the minimum number for a more linguistically advanced child; 100–150 utterances may be required for a reserved or language-delayed child.

There are advantages in collecting a continuous speech sample. Because the sampling procedure requires children to communicate much as they do in daily interactions, continuous speech is a more valid reflection of phonological ability. Another advantage is that this sampling procedure allows for multiple productions of sounds, which can reveal variability in production across lexical items. Finally, intelligibility can be estimated from a continuous sample, whereas it cannot be adequately determined from single words.

Disadvantages of continuous speech sampling were identified in Chapter 4. They include: (1) length of time required to collect, transcribe, and analyze a continuous speech sample; (2) reluctance of a reticent child to talk during the sampling procedure, resulting in a limited sample; and (3) production of unintelligible speech, for which the adult model is unknown. However, for the child with multiple errors, it is essential to sample continuous speech in order to have a varied enough corpus to describe the nature of the child's phonological system and identify deficits. Although the continuous sampling technique takes more time than a single-word articulation test, the results from a continuous speech sample provide the most representative information for analysis and therefore for selection of treatment goals. Two sampling procedures, an articulation test of some sort and a continuous speech sample, can be used together to obtain the most comprehensive corpus.

Recording the Sample

Audiotape recordings are essential for both types of articulation tests and continuous speech samples. It is difficult to impossible to accurately transcribe unintelligible continuous speech during collection of a sample. Even if the examiner is able to transcribe the productions of single words during the articulation test, it is important to be able to check the accuracy of the transcription later. In addition, transcription of complete words, rather than single segments, is important because it provides useful information about the effects of context within words (e.g., Nasal Assimilation: /mæmp/ for *lamp*). Because live transcription of whole words is difficult during sampling, the tape recording can supplement the transcription made during the sample. Important recording considerations outlined by Shriberg and Kwiatkowski (1980) include use of:

1. An external microphone placed 6–12 inches from the child's mouth for a good signal-to-noise ratio
2. A high-quality tape recorder and microphone that records a wide range of frequencies (20–20,000 Hz) for speech
3. High-quality, low-noise tape
4. A quiet setting, with a cloth or rug to muffle the noise of objects used to elicit the sample

Attention to the details of recording can make the difference in obtaining a high-quality sample that can be transcribed accurately.

Unintelligible Speech When collecting a sample from a child who is essentially unintelligible, it is helpful to repeat into the tape recorder any part of the child's utterance that is understood. If a second person is available, that person may write the utterances orthographically. These two techniques incorporate the situational context, which is not available during later transcription. When these techniques are used, speech that seems unintelligible initially can often be transcribed successfully. For the child who is almost completely unintelligible, it is necessary to supplement the continuous sample with single-word productions. Using the same words in both sampling conditions is helpful for making comparisons between single words and continuous speech. For example, the objects from the Assessment of Phonological Processes described earlier (Hodson, 1980) could be used to elicit the continuous sample.

Another technique for children who are difficult to understand is delayed imitation of words or sentences. Such a procedure is available in the Phonological Process Analysis (Weiner, 1979). In this procedure there are two levels of production. First, the child completes a sentence using a single word after the clinician's stimulus (e.g., "This is a fish" as the clinician points to fish. "Uncle Fred is catching a <u>fish</u>." Then the child responds with a phrase to a stimulus question, e.g., "What is Uncle Fred doing?" <u>Catching a fish</u> (Weiner, 1979). The stimuli allow the identification of <u>16</u> phonological processes in the child's speech. This procedure is useful when it is difficult to obtain a continuous speech sample, but the stimuli are limited in the speech they elicit. Other aspects of this procedure are reviewed by Dunn (1982).

Transcribing the Sample

When transcribing a sample, a decision must be made about the amount of phonetic detail that will be noted. For most substitutions, broad phonemic transcription is sufficient. For sound productions that cannot be represented by a standard phonemic symbol alone, narrow transcription using either diacritic symbols or phonetic symbols not found in adult English symbols is desirable. These symbols reflect: (1) coarticulation effects that sounds have on each other when they co-occur (e.g., lip-rounding of a consonant that co-occurs with a rounded vowel); or (2) productions that do not conform to adult English productions, e.g., a dentalized alveolar consonant, [d̪], or a voiced bilabial fricative, [β]. These symbols should be used when intelligibility is affected or when attention is drawn to a child's speech by non-English productions. If such productions are consistently and frequently used, they may be targets for remediation. For further information about narrow transcription, see Shriberg and Kent (1982), who discussed the clinical use of diacritics in detail. The diacritic symbols that we believe are most useful for disordered phonology are presented in Appendix A.

In summary, collection of a sample is a critical part of the assessment in terms of both the type of sample and the procedures of recording and transcription. The quality of the sample and its transcription determine the quality of the analysis that can be done and ultimately influences the decisions to be made about the adequacy of the child's phonological system.

Selection and Organization of Words for Analysis

Once the sample is transcribed, it is necessary to select and organize a subsample of words for analysis. The words selected must be organized in some fashion, e.g., alphabetized (Ingram, 1981) or arranged by sound class and word structure (Shriberg and Kwiatkowski, 1980). This step of organization is important because it permits the clinician to see patterns of production. Our preference for data organization is an adaptation of Shriberg and Kwiatkowski's coding sheet. Figure 6.1 is an example of our sheet; the words on the sheet were taken from the sample of the first child (DE) described below in the section on analysis (see Table 6.3).

The variables on the sheet are those that we have found to be important for making decisions about the child's phonological system. The first variable, sound class, displays consonants in a way that reveals patterns of errors (e.g., stopping of fricatives). One sheet is used for stops; a second sheet is used for nasals, glides, and liquids; and a third is used for fricatives and affricates. The second variable, word position, displays correct and incorrect sound productions that occur for initial, medial, or final word position (e.g., Final Consonant Deletion). The third variable, word structure, organizes words by singleton consonants (columns 1, 4, and 6 in Figure 6.1), consonant clusters and abutting consonants (columns 2, 5, and 7), and multisyllabic words (column 3, 4, 5, and 8). These sheets do not account for vowels; a similar organizational framework could be developed if an analysis of vowels were desired.

Typically 80–100 words are selected sequentially from the transcribed sample. Words should be selected to ensure that multiple opportunities for most consonants and a wide variety of word structures are included. Each word is coded by every consonant in the word. For example, DE produced the word *basket*, which has three stops: /b, k, t/. Therefore this word was entered in columns 3, 5, and 8 for the three consonants, respectively. Multiple entries of words provide extensive information but are time-consuming. If a partial analysis is desired, words can be coded by one or two variables, e.g.: (1) word position (initial); (2) a particular word structure (multisyllabic); or (3) a sound class (velar). In summary, we have found this framework effective for data organization because it makes patterns of errors obvious. For example, in Figure 6.1, it is readily apparent that in word-final position DE produced singleton labial and alveolar stops correctly and replaced velar stops with alveolar stops.

Name: DE
Age: 4;6

Sampling condition: *The Assessment of Phonological Processes*
Date of sampling: 11/24/82

	Initial			Medial		Final		
Stops	1. CV(C)	2. CⁿV(C)	3. Multisyllabic	4. -C-	5. -Cⁿ-	6. (C)VC	7. (C)VCⁿ	8. Multisyllabic
p	page [seɪʒ]	spoon [sũn] spring [swĩn]	paper ['fæfɚ]	open ['oɪtɛn] paper ['fæfɚ] zipper ['zɪpə]	airplane ['ɛɚsẽn]	cup [sʌp] rope [rop] soap [sop]	jump [ʒʌp]	makeup ['metap]
b	bed [bid] Bo [bo] book [but]	brown [bãn]	baseball ['bæbʌ] basket ['bæsɪt]	cowboy ['soboɪ]	baseball ['bæbʌ] football ['fʌtba] toothbrush ['tʰusrəʃ]	tub [sʌb]		
t	ten [zɛ̃n] tub [sʌb] two [tsu]	star [saʌ] stick [tʰɪ] string [swĩn] truck [tᶠʌt]	TV [sivi] television ['tsɛzĩn] toothbrush ['tʰusrəʃ] [tʃesrəʃ]	glitter ['zɪdə] scooter ['zʌdə] water ['waə]	football ['fʌtba] quarter ['tʃwʌdə]	hat [æt]	shirt [ʃɚt]	basket ['bæsɪt] minutes ['mĩnəz]

136

d	doll [daʌ]				screwdriver ['ʃudaɪbɚ] candle ['sæ̃ndl]	bed [bid] sled [sɛd]	and [ʌ] closed [sozd] hand [hæ̃n]	music ['musɪt]
k	couch [tʃautʃ] cup [sʌp]	Claus [sɔz] clothes [soz] closed [sozd] squirrel [swɛl]	candle ['sændl] coffee ['sɔsi] cowboy ['soboɪ] colors ['sʌzɚz] scooter ['zʌdɚ] screwdriver ['ʃudaɪbɚ]	makeup ['metʌp] wrecker ['wɛdɚ]	basket ['bæsɪt]	book [but] like [lɛt] Luke [zʌt] snake [set] stick [tʰɪ] truck [tʰʌt]	fork [sɔɪt]	
g	gun [zʌn]	glove [sʌz] green [wĩn, sĩn]	Christmas ['sɪtmʌs] quarter ['tʃwʌdɚ] glasses ['sæzɪz] glitter ['zɪdɚ]		Fall Guy [sʌ daɪ] finger ['fĩdɚ]	rug [wʌd]		

Figure 6.1 Data organization for selecting words for analysis.

137

Analysis of a Sample

Framework for Analysis

It is important to have a framework on which to base an analysis in order to ensure that all relevant aspects of the phonological system are considered. Such a framework was presented in Chapter 4; Table 6.1 summarizes the components of this framework. Two major types of analysis were described for analyzing children's data: independent analysis and relational analysis. This same framework is appropriate for phonologically disordered children for the following reasons. Description of production without reference to the adult form is important to show what segmental phones and syllable structures the child is capable of producing. Comparison of productions with the adult model is important in order to determine how closely the child is approximating the adult model. Discrepancies between the child and adult systems can be identified and used in conjunction with the description of production abilities when selecting treatment goals.

This framework is intended as a guideline for analysis. It may not be necessary to include each aspect in the analysis of speech of every phonologically disordered child. For example, it may be obvious from scanning the words selected for analysis that a child correctly produces consonants in word-final position. Therefore analysis of this aspect of the child's system would not be necessary.

In the Appendix of Chapter 4, we discussed the use of com-

Table 6.1 Framework for Analysis of Disordered Phonology

Independent Analysis of the Child's Productions	*Relational Analysis of the Child's Productions*
1. Inventory of phones: classified by word position and articulatory features	1. Inventory of sounds produced correctly and incorrectly: classified by word position and articulatory features
a. Single phones (consonants, vowels)	a. Single phones (consonants, vowels)
b. Clusters	b. Clusters
2. Inventory of word shapes which child produces	2. Sequential constraints
3. Sequential constraints	3. Phonological processes

puter programs to complete phonological analyses. Although saving time and increasing accuracy are attractive benefits, there are limitations in using computer-assisted analyses with phonologically disordered children. First, these children often have idiosyncratic processes, e.g., Glottal Replacement or Stops substituted for Glides. Although these substitutions would be identified, they would not be termed *processes* unless they were preprogrammed into the analysis. However, it would be difficult to impossible to anticipate all of the idiosyncratic processes that might occur in disordered speech. Second, other characteristics, particularly Sound Preference and Chronological Mismatch, require integration and comparison of different parts of the analysis for identification. For example, Sound Preference is identified when several consonants are replaced by one consonant or feature. At this point, there are no computer programs that can provide this type of post hoc analysis. Finally, disordered children often have distortions of a target phone, which must be coded with diacritics; as mentioned in Chapter 4, there are currently no programs that include diacritics. All of these examples show that: (1) characteristics of disordered phonology must be incorporated into computer programs; and (2) programs are not able to identify all relevant patterns in disordered speech. At best, computer-assisted analysis can perform only part of an analysis for phonologically disordered children.

Comparison of Analysis with Developmental Information

After completing an analysis of a child's segmental productions, the results are considered in relation to normal acquisition information. This comparison indicates: (1) if the child is acquiring the sound system within the expected age range; and (2) how the child's production and meaningful use of phonemes differ from the patterns of normal children. For example, if a 4-year-old child has correct production of liquids /l/ and /r/ but persists in using processes that normal children typically eliminate early, e.g., Final Consonant Deletion, this child's system differs from normally developing systems. As this example indicates, there is a need to use more developmental information than single-sound acquisition data (e.g., Templin, 1957). Other aspects of acquisition need to be considered when formulating a diagnosis. For example, in Chapter 2, information was presented relative to development of: (1) sound classes; (2) syllable shape; (3) sounds in relation to word position; and (4) types, occurrence, and elimination of phonological processes.

Integration of Analysis with Test Results

In order to determine the etiology of a phonological disorder, the results of the phonological analysis must be integrated with results from other tests. Table 6.2 presents seven supplementary test areas that are routinely included in a diagnostic evaluation of a phonological disorder. These areas are: (1) description of suprasegmental characteristics; (2) oral mechanism: structure and function; (3) stimulability; (4) hearing acuity and middle ear function; (5) speech perception; (6) expressive syntax; and (7) cognition. The table also presents references that provide a rationale for including these areas in an assessment of phonological disorders and guidelines for completing each evaluation. Disability in any of the seven areas may be related to a phonological disorder in one of two ways.

In some cases there may be a cause–effect relationship between the area of disability (e.g., hearing loss) and the phonological problem; in others, the disability may co-occur with a phonological disorder, without a cause–effect relationship. An unequivocal determination of the relationship between a supplementary area and phonological output is often impossible (Bernthal and Bankson, 1981; Winitz, 1969). However, difficulties in one or more of these areas often co-occur with a phonological disorder. For example, children with multiple phonological errors often exhibit problems encoding syntactic structures (Shriberg, 1982b). It is unclear whether the syntax problem causes the phonological problem or vice versa, or if the two problems are indicative of a broader-based language problem. However, regardless of whether the supplementary area causes or co-occurs with the phonological

Table 6.2 Areas for Supplementary Evaluation

Areas for Evaluation	References for Procedures
Suprasegmental characteristics	Shriberg and Kwiatkowski (1982a)
Oral mechanism structure and function	Mason and Simon (1977); St. Louis and Ruscello (1981)
Stimulability	Carter and Buck (1958); Madison (1979)
Speech perception	Locke (1980a,b)

Hearing
  a. Auditory acuity
  b. Impedance
	Martin (1981)

Expressive syntax	Miller (1981); Shriberg (1982b)
Cognition	Arthur (1952); Uzgiris and Hunt (1975); Westby (1980)

disorder, this information must be considered when forming decisions about etiology, management, and selection of treatment goals. A brief discussion is provided here about the first four areas (see above) because of the potential significance each area has for disordered phonology.

Suprasegmental Characteristics One of the most neglected areas of phonological assessment is suprasegmental characteristics. There are virtually no guidelines for assessing suprasegmentals or identifying difficulties that phonologically disordered children may have. Shriberg and Kwiatkowski (1982b) provided a rating scale for voice (pitch, loudness, quality) and rhythm (phrasing, stress, and rate) characteristics. They suggested listening to a recording of continuous speech and assigning a rating of 0 (normal), 1 (slight to pronounced deviations on less than 10–15% of the utterances in the sample), or 2 (slight to pronounced deviations on more than 10–15%). Their preliminary studies show that approximately two-thirds of the 43 children they studied were rated with a 1 or 2 on one or more of the six suprasegmental characteristics. Voice quality was most often rated as 2, but it is not known if the disordered children would actually differ from normal children on this characteristic. It was suggested that deviance with rate or stress may be more prevalent for children with motor speech involvement than for children with no apparent involvement (Shriberg and Kwiatkowski, 1982b). Until more is known about suprasegmental skills in disordered children, Shriberg and Kwiatkowski's procedure is a useful way to informally quantify this aspect of speech production.

Oral Mechanism: Structure and Function An examination of the *structure* of the oral mechanism includes observation of the structures at rest to determine if they seem adequate for speech production. Examination of the *function* of the oral mechanism includes observation of nonspeech movements (e.g., puckering the lips) and speech movements (rapid repetition of nonsense syllables, referred to as diadochokinesis). The purpose of the repeated movements is to determine if the rapid, ballistic movements required for speech can be achieved. This examination is typically a brief screening, rather than an in-depth evaluation. St. Louis and Ruscello (1981) suggested that the results of the screening should allow one of three judgments about the structure or function of the mechanism:

1. Normal, indicating that there are no obvious conditions that might interfere with speech

2. Referral to another professional (e.g., in case of suspected paralysis or velopharyngeal incompetence)
3. Further in-depth testing (e.g., in case of suspected oral apraxia or velopharyngeal incompetence)

These authors made an important point about the interpretation of the oral mechanism examination, noting that:

> There is an extreme range of normality in structure and function of the oral speech mechanism, and it is difficult to establish causal relationships between structural or functional deficits and a coexisting speech problem. (p. 7)

This caution reminds us that our role in assessment is one of careful observation and description, without labeling the child as having a "motor problem."

Stimulability A traditional part of phonological assessment is stimulability testing. This procedure evaluates the ability to correctly initiate error sounds after an auditory model and cues, which include instructions about placement of the articulators. Attention is often drawn to the visual model for placement and to the tactile sensations that accompany the positioning of the articulators. Sounds incorrectly produced during speech sampling are stimulated in words, nonsense syllables, or isolation. Our own clinical work has shown that stimulation that begins at the highest linguistic level (words) with the fewest number of cues (auditory only) provides the most information in the least amount of time. If a child is not successful at this level, additional cues can be added systematically at lower linguistic levels until success is achieved or it is determined that the child cannot produce the sound.

The correct responses that the child makes to stimulation reflect motoric ability to produce the sound, as well as adequate perceptual ability. Results of stimulability testing are used as both prognostic indicators and information for planning the treatment program. Correct responses to nonsense syllables are the best indicators that the child will spontaneously correct the sound (Carter and Buck, 1958; Farquhar, 1961). It is possible that success with stimulability is an indicator of readiness (Madison, 1979) and therefore is a useful tool for selecting phonemes to teach in treatment.

Speech Perception It is widely accepted that adequate auditory perception is essential for mastery of the phonological system. Phonologically disordered children are often thought to have problems with speech perception (Winitz, 1975). However, the exact nature of this perceptual deficit has not been determined. The deficit may involve: (1) speech sound discrimination; (2) identification of target phonemes in words; or (3) recognition and judgment of production errors. Traditionally, speech perception in phonologically disordered children has been assessed with general speech-sound discrimination tests (e.g., same–different tasks, as in Wepman's 1973 Auditory Discrimination Test) or with identification of phonemes in words presented with picture stimuli, (e.g., in the 1970 Goldman–Fristoe–Woodcock Test of Auditory Discrimination). These tests do not necessarily assess the sounds that children produce incorrectly. Locke (1980a,b) suggested that the only clinically relevant use of perceptual testing is evaluation of the child's productive errors because most phonologically disordered children do not have difficulty perceiving all sounds. Therefore perceptual testing should be limited to testing children's ability to differentiate between correct production and their own (incorrect) production of a target sound.

The remainder of this chapter provides sample analyses of the speech of two phonologically disordered children, ages 4;6 and 5;10. Both children were rated as severely disordered based on the percentage of consonants correct in their speech samples (47% and 33% correct, respectively) (Shriberg and Kwiatkowski, 1982b). However, they differed in their phonological characteristics. Therefore slightly different analysis procedures were used for the two samples. In both cases the children's productions are first described in terms of an independent analysis, then in terms of a relational analysis. The analyses are then integrated with developmental information and supplementary testing results.

Description of Analyses

The analyses were completed with certain guidelines in mind. First, a phonological analysis is completed in detail only for children with multiple errors; children with few errors do not require such detailed analysis. For children with milder problems, analysis of only one or two components may be sufficient. Second, the analysis should facilitate selection of goals for treatment. Thus certain components would not be analyzed if they would not be selected for treatment. For example, if a child does not have vowel errors, detailed analysis of the vocalic system would not be performed. Third, the relative frequencies of production should be determined, so that the relevance of particular sound occurrences, errors, or phonological processes can be identified. For example, if the process Velar Fronting occurs in a child's speech, one would

Table 6.3 DE, Age 4;6: 89 Selected Words

Gloss	Transcription	Gloss	Transcription
airplane	'ɛɚ·sēn	minutes	'mīnəz
and	ʌ	money	'mʌ̃ni
baseball	'bæbʌ	mouth	maʊf
basket	'bæsɪt	music	'musɪt
bed	bid	nose	noz
Bo	bo	open	'otɛ̃n
book	bʊt	orange	'ozɛd
brown	bə̃n	page	sets̬
candle	'sændl̩	paper	'fæfɚ
chair	'sɛɚ	quarter	'tʃwʌdə
Christmas	'sɪtmʌs	rope	rop
Claus	sɔz	rough	rʌf
clothes	soz	rug	wʌd
closed	sozd	Santa	'sænə
coffee	'sɔsi	screwdriver	'ʃudaɪbɚ
couch	ts̬auts̬	scooter	'zʌdə
cowboy	'sobɔi	shirt	ʃɚt
colors	'sʌzɚz	shoe	su
cup	sʌp	sled	sɛd
doll	daʌ	snake	set
Fall Guy	sʌ daɪ	soap	sop
feather	'ts̬ɛdə	spoon	sūn
finger	'fĩndə	spring	swīn
fish	sɪs	squirrel	swɛl
flower	'flaʊə	star	saʌ
football	'fʌtba	stick	tʰɪ
fork	sɔɪt	string	swīn
four	foə	TV	sivi
glasses	'sæzɪz	television	'ts̬ɛzĩn
glitter	'zɪdə	ten	zɛ̃n
glove	sʌz	this	dīs
green	wīn, sīn	three	ri, tʰi
gun	zʌ̃n	thumb	zʌ̃m
hand	æ̃n	toothbrush	'tʰusrəʃ
hanger	hʌ̃n	truck	tʰʌt
hat	æt	tub	sʌb
horse	hos	two	ts̬ʊ
ice	aɪts	vase	bes
Joe	do	watch	wats̬
jump	ʒʌp	water	'waə
knife	naɪf	wrecker	'wɛdə
leaf	sif	yellow	'ts̬eə
like	let	yoyo	'jojo
Luke	zʌt	zipper	'zɪpə
makeup	'metəp		

want to know how frequently it could potentially occur, as well as how often it actually occurred, in order to determine if it occurred frequently enough to require treatment. Numerical quantification was not stressed in the analyses of normal children's samples because such children acquire the phonological system with little difficulty. However, for disordered children, quantification provides information for selection of treatment goals and a baseline from which to measure progress.

Sample I: DE, Age 4;6

DE was diagnosed as phonologically disordered based on the results of the analysis presented here and the supplementary information obtained from the diagnostic evaluation. DE was unintelligible, at times even to his parents. He was reluctant to talk during the evaluation, even with his mother present. He had few utterances that were more than one word in length. The words for analysis (Table 6.3) were based on spontaneous one- and two-word utterances produced during the evaluation and responses from the Assessment of Phonological Processes (Hodson, 1980). The independent analysis of DE's productions includes: (1) an inventory of vowels, consonants, and clusters; and (2) word shapes. The relational analysis includes: (1) an inventory of sounds used correctly and incorrectly; and (2) a phonological process analysis. An analysis of sequential constraints and contrastive phones was not completed because information about this component was available through inspection of the speech sample or other analyses.

Independent Analysis

Inventory of Vowels, Consonants, and Clusters The inventory of vowels, consonants, and clusters (Table 6.4) presents the phones occurring in DE's productions; they are listed according to initial, medial, and final word position and manner class. Within each manner class, the consonant phones are ordered from front to back for place features, and the voiceless member of any cognate pair is listed first, e.g., [p, b, t, d, k, g]. This organizational framework provides information about articulatory features produced. To be included in the inventory, a phone had to occur three times in a given word position; if it occurred once or twice it was marked with parentheses and was considered marginal in the analysis. Initial and final clusters are also presented in Table 6.4.

DE produced the front vowels [i, ɪ, ɛ, e, æ], central vowels [ʌ, ə], back vowels [u, ʊ, o, ɔ, a], and diphthongs [aɪ, aʊ]. He produced all consonant manner classes; stops and fricatives were the most frequent. All place features were produced except inter-dental and velar; alveolar productions occurred most frequently. Voiced and voiceless cognates occurred in all word positions. The

Table 6.4 Phonetic Inventory and Frequency of Occurrence of Vowels,[a] Consonants, and Consonant Clusters

		Word Position					
Manner Class		Initial		Medial		Final	
Vowels:	i, ɪ, ɛ, e, æ, ʌ, ə, u, ʊ, o, ɔ, a						
Diphthongs:	aɪ, aʊ						
Consonants							
Stop				(p)	1	p	5
		b	7	b	4	(b)	1
		t	4	t	4	t	9
		d	4	d	7	d	4
Fricative		f	4	(f)	1	f	4
				(v)	1		
		s	27	s	5	s	5
		z	7	z	4	z	6
		(ʃ)	2[b]				
		(ʒ)	1			(ʃ)	1
Affricate		t͜s	5			t͜s	5
Nasal		m	5	(m)	1	(m)	1
		(n)	2	n	5	n	12
Liquid		r	3	(r)	1	ɪ̆	3
		(l)	1	(ɚ)	1	(ɚ)	1
Glide		w	5				
		(j)	1	(j)	1		
		(h)	2				
Consonant Clusters							
/s/ + glide		sw	3				
Affricate + glide		(tʃw)	1				
Fricative + liquid		(fl)	1				
Fricative + obstruent						(zd)	1
Stop + fricative						(ts)	1
Nasal + stop				(nd)	1		
Liquid + obstruent						(ɚt)	1
						(ɚt)	1

[a]Frequency of occurrence of vowels is not presented because vowels were not the focus of analysis.

[b]Sounds that occurred fewer than three times were noted in parentheses.

phone [s] occurred most frequently in the sample (35 times), followed by [z] and [t] (17 times each). The manner, place, and voicing features that were produced occurred in all three word positions. In initial position, 10 phones occurred at least three times, whereas six occurred in medial and nine in final word position. Thirteen other phones were produced once or twice in at least one position. No velar consonants occurred in the sample, and there were few voiced fricatives in word-initial position. In summary, DE produced a wide variety of articulatory features in a variety of phonetic contexts. Cluster production was very limited relative to the variety of phones produced as single consonants.

Syllable and Word Shape The word shapes produced by DE are described relative to their C (consonant) and V (vowel or diphthong) structures. DE produced some complex word shapes, e.g., 'CVCCVC. However, the most frequently occurring word shapes had a relatively simple structure:

CV	7
CVV	5
CVC	38
'CVCV	13
'CVCVC	6

He produced consonant clusters in all word positions, but his predominant word shapes did not include clusters. *Syllable* shapes were similar to word shapes in that there were several different ones, but the predominant shapes were simple, e.g., CV and CVC.

Relational Analysis

Comparison of Phones with Adult Form The comparison of phones with adult form identified errors and correct productions of each phone and cluster that was attempted (Table 6.5). For singleton consonants, the stops /b/ and /d/ were accurately produced. For /p,t,k,g/ other sounds were substituted; half of these substitutions (16/30) were fricatives, e.g., [s] for /t/. For fricatives, /s/ and /z/ were the most accurate; /f/ and /ʃ/ were the only other fricatives that were ever correct. No affricates were correct; however, DE produced [t͜s] as a substitution several times. The nasals /m/ and /n/ were always correct, but /ŋ/ was never correct. The liquids /l/ and /r/ were correct half the time, only in initial position; /ɝ/ and /ɚ/ were correct in medial and final positions. For glides, DE was most consistently correct with /w/; /j/ and /h/ were correct

Table 6.5 Correct and Incorrect Productions Classified by Word Position

Target Phoneme	Initial		Medial		Final	
	Correct/Total	Production	Correct/Total	Production	Correct/Total	Production
p	0/2	s,f	1/3	t,f	3/3	
b	5/5		2/2		1/1	
t	1/6	s,z,tʃ	1/5	d,r	2/2	
d	1/1		—		2/2	
k	0/2	s,tʃ	0/5	p,s,t	0/6	t
g	0/2	z/d	0/1	d	0/1	d
f	3/7	s,tʃ	0/1	s	3/3	
v	0/1	b	0/2	b, ø	0/1	z
θ	0/2	z	—		0/1	f
ð	0/1	d	—		—	
s	2/2		1/4	s,z,ø	3/4	tʃ
z	1/1		0/1	s	4/4	
ʃ	1/2	s	—		1/2	s
ʒ	—		—		—	
tʃ	0/1	s	—		0/1	s
dʒ	0/2	ʒ	—		0/1	tʃ
m	6/6		1/1		1/1	
n	2/2		4/4		7/7	
ŋ	—		0/2	n	0/2	n
l	1/3	s,z	0/2	z,ø	0/3	ø
r	2/4	w	0/2	z,ø	0/2	vowel
ɚ	—		1/1	ø	4/13	ø, vowel
w	4/4		0/1	ø	—	
j	1/2	tʃ	0/1		—	
h	2/4	ø	1/1		—	
Total	32/62 (52%)		12/38 (32%)		31/60 (52%)	

148

50% of the time in initial position. DE produced all place features correctly except interdental and velar. Alveolar phones were substituted frequently for other phones, e.g., [s] for /f/ and [t] for /k/. For the cognate pairs that were produced, voicing distinctions were usually accurate.

In summary, DE was able to produce phones in the following manner:

1. Always correct: b,d,m,n (4)
2. Intermittently correct: p,t,f,s,z,ʃ,l,r,w,j,h (11)
3. Never correct: k,g,v,θ,ð,ʒ,tʃ,ʤ,ŋ (9)

For the phones that were intermittently correct, there were often two or three different context-free substitutions (i.e., substitutions that were not conditioned by the sounds of the neighboring phonetic context). For example, /l/ was produced correctly, deleted, or substituted with [s] and [z]. Therefore few phones were consistently correct, and there was variability in the phones that were substituted for the target phone. When considering correct matches by word position, the results were initial 52%, medial 32%, and final 52%. Error patterns were similar across all word positions, with the medial position being less accurate than other word positions.

DE attempted many words with clusters. However, he produced only one cluster correctly in initial position: [fl]. For other initial clusters with /l/ and /r/, he deleted the liquid and produced the remaining phone correctly (e.g., [b] for /br/) or substituted another phone (e.g., [s] for /gr/). For /s/ clusters, DE usually retained the [s] and deleted the other member, e.g., [s] for /sn/. In final position, there was one correct cluster: [zd]. Other clusters were reduced to one member or were deleted: /mp, nd, rk, rs/. DE's vowel production was generally accurate. He had occasional substitutions (e.g., [æ] for /e/ and [ʌ] for /u/), but there were no consistent errors.

Phonological Processes The purpose of a phonological process analysis is to identify error patterns that affect general word structures or sound classes. The processes described in Chapters 2 and 5 that characterize normal and phonologically disordered children were used as the basis for the analysis. Table 6.6 presents the result of the analysis. The potential and actual occurrence of each process was identified; comparison of potential occurrence relative to actual occurrence is essential to determine the relevance of a process in a child's system. A percentage of occurrence for each process was computed.

Table 6.6 Phonological Processes: Actual, Potential, and Percentage of Occurrence

Phonological Process	Actual/ Potential Occurrences	Percentage	Distributional Patterns
Syllable Structure			
Deletion			
Initial position	1/60	2	h
Medial position	5/40	13	s,ɾ,k,w,l
Final position	3/53	6	k,l
Weak Syllable Deletion	1/34	3	Medial, unstressed syllable
Cluster Reduction	33/40	83	All positions and sound classes
Substitution			
Velar Fronting	14/34	41	All positions
Stopping	8/62	13	All positions
Depalatalization	7/11	64	Initial, final position
Gliding	5/30	17	Initial, medial position
Vocalization	10/28	36	Final position
Assimilation[a]			
Fricative	6	—	—
Alveolar	2	—	—

[a]Potential occurrences were not identified because assimilation of one sound to another could occur an incalculable number of times.

The processes are grouped by major type. The first type, syllable structure processes, represents sound changes that simplify the syllabic structure of the target word. DE was able to maintain syllable structure well, except for the production of clusters. Clusters were typically reduced to one member; the description of correct and incorrect cluster production was provided in the previous section.

In substitution processes, one class of sounds is substituted for another. As seen in Table 6.6, the occurrence of these processes ranged from 11 to 64%. These percentages must be viewed in perspective with DE's other errors. Processes accounted for only certain sound changes. Other errors, including idiosyncratic processes, also occurred in DE's speech. For example, Velar Fronting is the substitution of alveolars /t,d,n/ for velars /k,g,ŋ/, respectively. For DE, Velar Fronting occurred 41% of the time; however, the remaining attempts at velar productions were never correct. Instead, velars were deleted or substituted with other alveolars ([s,z,ts̺]). This example shows that process analysis can be misleading if the results are not considered in conjunction with other errors. The processes Stopping, Depalatalization, and Gliding were similar to Velar Fronting; in addition to the occurrence of the process, there were: (1) a few correct productions of the target phones; (2) deletions; and (3) several substitutions of [s,z,ts]. For Vocalization, the target sounds were correct or deleted when not substituted by a vowel. These productions are described in more detail above.

In assimilation processes, sounds become more similar to another within the word. There were eight words that may have been affected by assimilation:

coffee	'sɔsi
colors	'sʌzɚz
fish	sɪs
leaf	sif
page	sets̮
paper	'fæfɚ
open	'otɛ̃n
orange	'ozɛd

The assimilation processes described in Chapter 2 did not occur, e.g., Velar, Labial, Nasal Assimilation. The first six words above involve Fricative Assimilation because a target sound changed to a fricative. These sound changes may not have been assimilations. There were similar substitutions for these sounds (/k,f,l,ʃ,p/) when they occurred in words without fricatives, e.g., [ʃʌ] for *fall* and ['ɛɚsẽn] for *airplane*. However, because there was another fricative in the word, the fricative substitution may have been more likely. The last two words involve changes to alveolar production: [t] for /p/ and [z] for /r/. They may have occurred as a way to simplify the production by maintaining the same place of articulation throughout the word. In fact, all of the above words except *leaf* have the same place of articulation. Assimilation was not prevalent but may have been used occasionally as a means to simplify a complex production.

Idiosyncratic Processes DE had one idiosyncratic process, referred to as Sound Preference. He substituted the consonants [s,z,ts̮] for /p,t,k,g,f,v,θ,ð,tʃ,ʤ,j,r,l/ at least once. It was not predictable which of the three phones would be substituted for some target phones, e.g., [s,z,ts̮] for /t/. The Sound Preference was characterized by the articulatory features [alveolar] and [stridency]. The preference occurred in all word positions but it was more prevalent in initial position.

In addition to Sound Preference, DE exhibited an unusual pattern in his speech. He correctly produced some later developing phones (e.g., /s,z,ɚ/) while continuing to have difficulty with some phones that are typically mastered early, e.g., stops. This unusual co-occurrence of correct and error productions is referred to as Chronological Mismatch (Grunwell, 1981).

Phonemic Contrasts A final consideration about DE's segmental productions is the occurrence of phonemic contrasts. DE's ability to maintain contrasts among sounds and sound classes seemed to be in a state of flux. That is, contrasts were maintained in some words but not others. For example, /w/ and /r/ were not consistently contrasted because of the phonological process Gliding. Other contrasts lacking in initial position were between: (1) voiced and voiceless obstruents; (2) velars and alveolars (due to Velar Fronting); (3) stops and fricatives (due to fricative substitutions); and (4) singleton consonants and consonant clusters (due to Cluster Reduction). Other place and manner substitutions were maintained. Final contrasts were similar to those in initial position. This discussion of contrasts is not meant to be exhaustive but is presented to show how the analysis can be used to compare the adult phonemic system with that of the child.

Summary of Analyses When considering DE's system, it was seen that he produced all vowels, all consonant manner classes, and all places of articulation except interdental and velar. There were many phones in his repertoire, but several of them occurred infrequently. These marginal phones may have been emerging or may not have occurred in the sample of words selected. DE's productions were primarily alveolar fricatives and stops; a few non-English phones or sequences occurred, e.g., [ts̬] and [tʃw]. The inventory was similar across all three word positions. DE produced a large variety of word shapes. The majority of the productions were monosyllabic; CVC shapes occurred most frequently.

When comparing DE's system to the adult phonemic system, his vowels were generally accurate. Few consonant phonemes were consistently correct in any word position. Phonological process analysis revealed that substitutions accounted for most of his errors. Some substitutions were accounted for by the processes Velar Fronting, Gliding, Depalatalization, and Vocalization. The remaining substitutions were accounted for by DE's substitution of alveolar fricatives and affricates [s,z,ts̬].

Comparison of Analysis Results with Developmental Information

There is information from acquisition of consonants that suggest that a 4-year-old child can produce the majority of sounds correctly (Sander, 1972) and has eliminated most phonological processes (Hodson and Paden, 1981). When referring to Table 2.3 (customarily produced and mastered consonants) 4-year-old children customarily produced 21 consonants (all but /θ,ð,ʒ/). However, DE customarily produced only 11 sounds. When considering consonants that are correctly produced by 90% of normal 4-year-old children, there are 11: /p,b,d,k,g,m,n,f,w,j,h/. However, DE consistently and correctly produced only four consonants: /b,d,m,n/. Thus DE's consonant production was considerably below that of a normal 4;6-year-old. His performance in terms of number of sounds customarily and accurately produced was more like that of a 3-year-old.

Many clusters are produced consistently by 4-year-old children in both initial and final position (Table 2.5). DE was clearly delayed in cluster production. Although he did produce clusters, he rarely did so with any frequency or accuracy. When comparing singleton to cluster production, DE was less accurate on clusters than on singletons. His phonetic inventory included the singletons needed to pronounce the basic clusters (e.g., /stop + liquid/, /s + nasal or stop/), but he did not do so.

As mentioned earlier, normal 4-year-old children have usually eliminated most phonological processes by age 4, so that errors occur for isolated sounds and not classes or word structures. DE had only three processes that occurred more than 40% of the time: Cluster Reduction, Velar Fronting, and Depalatalization. However, he had problems with: (1) velar, palatal, and interdental place features; (2) affricate and liquid manner classes; and (3) voicing features. DE differed from normal and other disordered children because typical processes did not account for the majority of his errors.

There was one idiosyncratic process, Sound Preference, that accounted for many of DE's errors. The widespread substitution of the alveolar fricatives and affricate ([s,z,ts̲]) neutralized many potential contrasts. The substitution of the stridency feature for other manner features has been described for disordered children (Edwards, 1980b; Ingram, 1976; Weiner, 1981a) but not normal children. Finally, these substitutions were variable; all three phones were substituted for some of the target consonants. The combination of the unusual substitutions, the variability, and the neutralization of contrasts all resulted in speech that was highly unintelligible.

In summary, DE had a phonological system that was below expectation for a child of 4;6. He was performing in some ways like a normal 3-year-old, but his prevalent use of the stridency feature set him apart from normal and other disordered children. His phonological disorder was considered severe based on a comparison with developmental information.

Integration of Analysis Results with Test Results

In addition to the speech sample that was collected and administration of the Assessment of Phonological Processes (Hodson, 1980), other areas were evaluated to determine their possible relationship to the phonological disorder. Suprasegmental characteristics (voice and rhythm) were informally observed. It was difficult to draw any conclusions because DE spoke primarily in single-word utterances. Stress for individual words was appropriate, and pitch and intensity seemed accurate. A cursory examination of the oral mechanism suggested normal structure and function; however, DE was not willing to cooperate for a more comprehensive examination. His ability to produce many sounds in a variety of word structures supported the hypothesis that he was able to coordinate motor movements adequately, but further testing was recommended to confirm this.

Hearing acuity was within normal limits based on a hearing screening of each ear at 15 dB ISO for frequencies between 250 and 8,000 Hz. However, DE had a history of chronic middle ear infections, which continued to be a problem for him at the time of the evaluation. It was suspected that the phonological disorder was related to fluctuating hearing thresholds. Speech perception was not evaluated.

DE scored below age level on the Peabody Picture Vocabulary Test—Revised (Dunn, 1981), a measure of single-word receptive vocabulary; this performance may have been below his actual ability, because he participated in the evaluation reluctantly. He responded appropriately to instructions presented auditorily. Expressive language skills were impossible to evaluate thoroughly because of his poor intelligibility and his reluctance to talk. On imitative items from the Carrow Elicited Language Inventory (Carrow, 1974), DE omitted words, syllables, and grammatical morphemes, which suggested that he may have had difficulty producing structures that were syntactically complex.

Diagnostic Statement

It was concluded that DE had a severe phonological disorder because of: (1) poor intelligibility; (2) limited repertoire of consistently correct consonant production; and (3) idiosyncratic Sound Preference, which neutralized contrasts. Etiology for the disorder was undetermined. However, the chronic middle ear problems may have contributed to the disorder. There was a possibility that DE had a language disorder that incorporated other components of the linguistic system in addition to phonology. Recommendations for management of the disorder included: (1) enrollment in treatment for remediation of the phonological disorder; (2) additional testing of language abilities as part of the treatment; and (3) immediate management and elimination of the chronic middle ear infections by an otolaryngologist.

Sample II: BC, Age 5;10

A second case illustrates the phonological system of another disordered child. Although her disorder was also diagnosed as severe, its patterns were quite different from those of DE.

BC was unintelligible when seen for a diagnostic evaluation. The continuous speech sample used for the following analysis was collected during an interactive play situation in a clinical setting. Approximately 150 utterances were produced, and 110 words were selected from these utterances for analysis (Table 6.7). The first analysis is the independent analysis of the child's productions, and the second is the relational analysis.

Independent Analysis

Inventory of Vowels, Consonants, and Clusters Initial, medial, and final phones in BC's productions are shown in Table 6.8. To be included, phones must have occurred three or more times; sounds that occurred once or twice are included in parentheses as marginal phones. Consonant clusters are also shown in the table. It can be seen from Table 6.8 that BC produced an extremely limited number of consonant phones. She consistently produced only stops and nasals that had labial or alveolar place of production; the phones [t,d,n] occurred most frequently. Production of phones in medial and final position was more limited than initial position. BC pro-

Table 6.7 BC, Age 5;10: 110 Selected Words

Gloss	Transcription	Gloss	Transcription
all right	'ɔwaɪ	give	dɪ
animal	'ænə	go	do
another	'n:ʌdə	hair	ɛə
anything	'ɪnɪtēn	helicopter	'ʌlətɔɪ
Batman	'bæʔmæn	happening	'æʔɪnə̄n
bed	bɛ:	hello	hɛ'do
bicycle	'baɪtɪʔə	hiding	aīn
big	bɪʔ	him	ī:ə
bottle	'ba:ɾo	home	ō:
bring	bwī:	house	a:
broke	bo:	into	īn'tu
broom	bū:	just	də
brought	bɔʔ	knife	naɪ
brush	bʌ:	ladder	'ædə
brushing	'bʌʔīn	leave	li
bus	bʌ	little	'tʰɪrl̩
bye	baɪ	like	aɪʔ
camera	'tʰǣ:mo:	medicine	'mɛdī ʔīn
cap	tʰæ	mama	'māma
car	tʰɔ:	many	'mīni
catch	tʰɛʔ	not	naʔ
catching	'tʰɛʔīn	nobody	'nobəʔə
caught	tʰɔʔ	okay	o'te
chair	tʰɛ:	other	'ʌdə
chicken	'tʰɪʔīn	pick	pʰɪʔ
choochoo	'tʰutu	picking	'pʰīʔɪn
climb	tʰāɪn	play	pʰe
cracker	'dæʔjɪʔ	Playdoh	'pwedo
cup	tʰʌ	place	pʰe
cutting	'tʰʌʔīn	put	pʰʊt
doctor	'da:ʔI	putting	'pʰīʔn̩
dolly	'da:wi	radio	'eio
don't	dō ʔ	riding	'aɪīn
donkey	'dɔ̄ʔi	sack	tʰæ
down	tʰaʔ	school	kʰu:
dress	dɛ:	send	tʰīn
drink	tʰɪ	shoe	tʰu:
drinking	'tʰiʔīn	shot	tʰaʔ
elephant	'ʌdətə̄n	sit	tʰɪʔ
empty	'īmpɪ	sleeping	'tʰiʔn̩
end	ī	some	tʰʌ
fine	tʰaɪ:	somebody	'tʰʌ̄mbaɪ
fire	'paɪjə	spoon	pu:
fireman	'paɪjəmæn	stair	tʰɛə
firetruck	'paɪjətəʔ	superman	'tʰuʔtəmæn
fish	tʰɪ	sweeping	'tʰiʔn̩
fishing	'tʰīʔɪn	telephone	'tʰɛdəto:
Frank	dē:nʔ	that	dæʔ
get	dɪʔ	then	dī:n
giraffe	dæ:	there	dɛ:

Table 6.7 (*continued*)

Gloss	Transcription	Gloss	Transcription
thing	tʰēn	we	wi
train	tʰēn	when	wī
too	tʰu	with	ɪʔ
up	ʌʔ	yeah	jæ
water	'ɔɾə	you	ju

duced three consonant clusters, [bw, pw, mp], as well as all the vowels of English.

Syllable and Word Shapes BC produced more than 24 word shapes, some of which were three syllables in length. However, more than half of the words were monosyllabic. The most prevalent word shapes were CV (34) and CVC (22). Syllable shapes were simple and included V, CV, VC, CVC, CCV, and CVCC. By far the most common shape was CV.

Relational Analysis

Comparison of Phones with Adult Form BC's productions of singleton consonants and clusters were compared to the adult form. From Table 6.9 it can be seen that five phones were consistently correct in initial position: [p,b,t,m,n]. In medial and final position, [m] and [n] were the only consistently correct phones. There were infrequent correct productions of a few other phones: [d,l,w,j,h]. For the phones that BC did not produce, she consistently substituted [t] or [d] in initial position; in other word positions she substituted either [t], [d], or [ʔ], or deleted the consonant. There was some variability between [t,d,ʔ] and the deletions, but overall BC was very consistent in her productions. Only one cluster, medial

Table 6.8 Phonetic Inventory: Initial, Medial, and Final Position

Manner	Inventory by Word Position		
	Initial	Medial	Final
Consonants			
Stop	p b t d (k)ª	(p) (b) t d	(t)
Nasal	m n	m n	n
Liquid	(l)		(l)
Glide	(w) (j) (h)	(w)	
Clusters	pw, bw	mp	

ªSounds that occurred fewer than three times are noted in parentheses.

Table 6.9 Correct Productions Classified by Word Position

Percent of Correct Productions	Initial	Medial	Final
100	p,b,t,m,n	m,n	n
50	d	t	
Produced correctly at least once	k,l,w,j,h	p,b,d,n,l	t,l

[mp], was produced correctly in the sample. For vowels, BC correctly produced the adult target in most words.

Phonological Processes BC had several error patterns that affected an entire class of sounds or word structures; these simplifications constituted a phonological process. The results of the analysis are presented in Table 6.10 in terms of the potential, actual, and percentage of occurrence. The first group, syllable structure processes, reveals that BC simplified adult word structure by deleting consonants, primarily in final word position and consonant clusters. These deletions resulted in a predominance of CV syllable shapes. All sound classes were affected by these processes.

BC produced no velar, fricative, or affricate consonants. The absence of these sound classes is represented by the substitution process Velar Fronting (49% occurrence) and Stopping (72% occurrence). The consonants [d] and [t] were the predominant substitutions for the processes. When the velars, fricatives, and affricates were not fronted or stopped, they were deleted or replaced by a glottal stop. The liquid class was also rarely correct. There was a tendency to delete initial /l/ and /r/ and to delete or to substitute [d] in medial position. The process of Vocalization occurred in 50% of the final productions; otherwise the liquids were deleted.

BC had four productions that were examples of Alveolar Assimilation:

elephant	ˈʌdətən
telephone	ˈtɛdəto
Superman	ˈtuʔtəmæn
little	ˈtɪrl̩

These assimilations resulted in a single place of articulation in all of the words except *Superman*. However, the change of /l/ and /f/ to alveolar stops in the first two words may have been substitutions, because [d] was substituted for /l/ and [t] for /f/ in other words (e.g., *hello* and *fine* Table 6.7). A few of BC's productions were accounted for by idiosyncratic processes, which are described below.

Table 6.10 Phonological Processes: Actual, Potential, and Percentage of Occurrence

Phonological Process	Actual/ Potential Occurrences	Percentage	Distributional Patterns
Syllable structure			
Deletion			
Initial position	14/78	18	l,r,h,w
Medial position	12/74	16	All sound classes
Final position	44/69	65	All sound classes
Weak Syllable Deletion	3/48	6	
Cluster Deletion	4/30	13	Final clusters
Cluster Reduction	23/30	77	All positions and sound classes
Substitution			
Velar Fronting	18/37	49	Primarily initial position
Stopping	36/50	72	Initial, medial position
Gliding	2/14	14	Medial position
Vocalization	9/18	50	Final position
Glottal Replacement	18/74	24	Medial position
Assimilation[a]			
Alveolar	4	—	—

[a]Potential occurrences were not identified because assimilation of one sound to another could occur an incalculable number of times.

Idiosyncratic Processes In Chapter 5 phonologically disordered children were described as demonstrating patterns of errors which infrequently occur in normal children. BC had two such processes, as seen in Table 6.10. Initial Consonant Deletion occurred in only 18% of the possible productions. However, it is noteworthy that liquids /l,r/ and glides /w,h/ were the only consonants deleted. Glottal Replacement occurred in 24% of the medial productions. When these productions are combined with medial deletions (16% occurrence) it can be seen that 40% of the medial consonants were not maintained.

Phonemic Contrasts BC's ability to maintain phonemic distinctions was severely reduced owing to the errors described above. In initial position, she maintained voicing contrasts, as well as contrasts among labial and alveolar stops and nasals. There was a lack of contrast between: (1) stops, fricatives, and affricates; (2) velar and alveolar stops; and (3) singleton consonants and clusters. In final position there was essentially no contrast due to widespread final consonant deletion. These examples do not describe all the difficulties with phonemic contrasts, but they do illustrate that BC did not seem to be aware or capable of maintaining distinctions among words. In fact, BC had such a limited inventory of sounds and word structures that many of her words were produced in the same way, resulting in several homophonous forms. For example, she produced [tʌ] for *cup* and *some* and [dɛ:] for *dress* and *there*. In all, there were 15 homophonous forms, representing 32 words, or almost one-third of the words selected for analysis. BC's productions of these homophonous forms, and in fact all words, were highly consistent.

Summary BC had a very limited repertoire of phones that she produced correctly. The correct phones (labial and alveolar stops and nasals) represented a limited set of features. Place features that were essentially absent included interdental, labiodental, palatal, and velar. Strident, liquid, and glide manner classes were not included consistently in her repertoire. Most words were produced with alveolar sounds because of: (1) correct production of [t,d,n]; (2) substitution of [t] or [d] for fricatives, affricates, and velars; and (3) deletion of many nonalveolar consonants. The deletions resulted in a predominance of CV syllable structures.

The phonological processes that occurred frequently in BC's sample were those that have been used to characterize normal and disordered phonology. When a process was not used, the consonant was usually deleted. BC's speech was not characterized by frequent occurrence of unusual processes. She did not have a large enough repertoire of sounds to maintain contrasts among words; this resulted in the production of many homophonous forms. BC's speech patterns were strikingly predictable; she showed little variability across different productions of the same words.

Comparison of Analysis with Developmental Information

BC's repertoire of phones was similar to that of a child 2–3 years old. She persisted in using phonological processes that are usually eliminated or greatly reduced by age 3;0, including Final Consonant Deletion, Stopping, Velar Fronting, and Vocalization. Unlike many severely disordered children, there were not frequent occurrences of idiosyncratic processes. She also did not demonstrate Chronological Mismatch, which is the correct production of consonants that tend to develop later (e.g., /l/ and /r/) concurrent with incorrect production of early-developing consonants (e.g., nasals). BC's speech patterns suggest that her phonological acquisition was similar to that of a very young normal child.

Integration of Analysis with Test Results

Other testing and analyses were completed to determine possible relationships between other variables and the phonological disorder. Informal observation of suprasegmental characteristics (pitch, loudness, and quality) indicated that voice quality was appropriate. Rate of speech was rapid, and BC's utterances sounded staccato owing to the frequent deletions and glottal replacements. Word stress was appropriate. An oral mechanism examination revealed structures and function that seemed adequate for speech. Production of both speech and nonspeech movements was slow but regular. BC had difficulty imitating the phones [k,g,f,s,ʃ] in any word position. However, she was successful in producing the phones at the nonsense syllable level after several trials of being presented with visual and tactile cues.

A hearing evaluation revealed normal hearing acuity. BC had a series of chronic middle ear infections from 5 months to 4 years of age. Since that time, infections had not recurred. Speech perception was not evaluated.

At the time of data collection, BC's receptive language skills, as measured by the Peabody Picture Vocabulary Test—Revised (Dunn, 1981) and the Test of Auditory Comprehension of Language (Carrow, 1973), were 6 months below age level. Expressive language skills were not formally evaluated because of poor intelligibility. BC omitted function words and morphological inflections in conversational speech. Mean length of utterance (MLU) from the continuous sample was 3.07, which was approximately 3 years below the expected MLU for a child almost 6 years old (Miller, 1981).

Diagnostic Statement

BC was diagnosed as having a severe phonological disorder based on: (1) poor intelligibility; (2) limited repertoire of consonants produced; (3) persistence of phonological processes; and (4) lack of phonemic contrasts. The etiology of the disorder was undetermined. Oral motor skills seemed delayed, but BC was capable of imitating speech movements; therefore apraxia of speech was considered unlikely. Chronic middle ear infections may have contributed to the disorder. In addition, there was a strong possibility that BC had a language problem in conjunction with the phonological disorder. Recommendations for management of the disorder included: (1) enrollment in treatment for the phonological disorder; (2) selection of phonological treatment goals and activities that would facilitate production of grammatical forms that BC omitted; and (3) evaluation of expressive language abilities as intelligibility improved.

Comparison of DE's and BC's Analyses

In order to place the phonological analyses of DE and BC into a broader perspective of disordered phonology, the two analyses are compared, first in terms of similarities and then in terms of differences. DE and BC were similar in that their disorders were both rated as *severe* based on the computation of a percentage of correct consonants (Shriberg and Kwiatkowski, 1982b). Both children were considered highly unintelligible by all listeners in their environments. Other *similarities* included:

1. Multiple errors when comparing their productions with the adult form
2. Few productions of consonant clusters
3. CV and CVC as the predominant word shapes
4. Difficulty in maintaining phonemic contrasts

The difficulty with contrasts seemed to stem from different causes. BC lacked contrasts because she had such a limited repertoire of phones with which to achieve contrasts; on the other hand, DE had a larger phonetic repertoire but did not consistently use it to distinguish among sound classes. *Differences* other than the use of contrasts included:

1. Number of phones, with DE producing many more phones than BC
2. Complexity of syllable and word shape, with DE producing more complex shapes
3. Occurrence of processes, with BC having predominant occurrence of processes that typify normal and disordered children, whereas DE had noticeably fewer occurrences of these processes
4. Idiosyncratic processes, with DE demonstrating a Sound Preference and a Chronological Mismatch, whereas BC had limited occurrence of such processes

5. Variability, with DE having considerable variability and BC having little

In sum, although both children had severe phonological disorders, the characteristics they manifested were quite different. These two children illustrate the striking differences that occur among children; their phonological patterns also suggest that very different remediation approaches would be required for each child.

Selection of Treatment Goals

The third objective of assessment is to select goals for the child who is enrolled in treatment. In order to illustrate this objective, treatment goals were selected for BC. The goals and the rationale for each are presented in Table 6.11.

Table 6.11 Treatment Goals for BC

Goal	Rationale
1. Increase repertoire of sounds in inventory. Focus for stimulation: a. Velar /k,ŋ/ b. Fricative /s,f,h/ c. Liquid /l/ Word position: initial and final	1. To provide a variety of features from all sound classes as alternatives to alveolar stops and nasals. The sounds were chosen because they occurred in the sample (/k,h,l/) or represent features that BC produced (/ŋ,s,f/).
2. Produce sounds correctly in word-final position. Focus: /p,b,t,d,n/	2. To expand the existing repertoire to other word positions. This goal would begin to eliminate the process of final consonant deletion and reduce homophonous forms.
3. Contrast sounds in final position of minimal-pair words. Focus: a. Sounds in goal 2 b. Sounds in goal 1	3. To illustrate the necessity of final consonants for accurate communication. (Production ability is a prerequisite for this goal.)
4. Produce sequences of two consonants. Focus: a. Initial /stop + l/ and /s + nasal/ clusters b. Final /nasal + stop/ clusters	4. To increase the complexity of syllable shapes in order to approximate the adult words attempted. The sounds were chosen because of the singleton and cluster consonants in BC's sample and according to clusters that are acquired first (Templin, 1957; Hodson and Paden, 1983).

The focus of the goals was to increase:

1. The phonetic inventory
2. *Correct* production and contrastive use of phones in word-final position
3. The complexity of syllables through production of initial and final clusters

Conclusions

This chapter has described assessment procedures that focus on data collection, phonological analysis, and integration of normative data and other test results with the phonological analysis. The framework for phonological analysis involves description of a child's productions through independent and relational analyses. This approach to assessment is based on the premise that clinicians make decisions about what is appropriate for a child at each step of assessment. A great deal of detail has been presented in this discussion to illustrate the kinds of decisions that can be made and the appropriate use of the information derived from such an analysis. As the clinician gains experience, the various analyses can be shortened or modified to serve the needs of the child. For example, only one or two word positions might be analyzed, and only certain processes might be identified, as indicated by the child's sample.

Some readers may believe that the analysis procedures described in this chapter are too time-consuming. They will argue that the same information can be derived from traditional articulation testing and analysis. Our response is that severely disordered children require a comprehensive description of their systems so that we can most effectively meet the objectives identified at the beginning of this chapter: (1) to determine if there is a phonological disorder and to possibly identify its etiology; (2) to make recommendations for management; and (3) to make suggestions for treatment goals. Only an in-depth analysis, integrated with other test results and normative data, can provide that information.

Chapter 7

Treatment of Disordered Phonology

During the last decade interest in phonological disorders has focused on the application of phonological concepts to treatment. These concepts involve consideration of speech production in relation to the linguistic system, so that more abstract phonological units (e.g., distinctive features or phonological processes) are the basic unit for treatment. The objective of remediation based on phonological concepts is to assist the child in acquiring the adult phonological system. The techniques focus on teaching meaningful concepts (e.g., that sounds contrast meaning) rather than on production practice. This chapter describes the application of phonological concepts to treatment. Application of distinctive features and phonological processes is discussed, as well as variables related to management of a treatment session. The variables include: (1) linguistic content; (2) the structure of a treatment session; (3) remediation techniques; (4) definition of a correct response and criteria for sound mastery; and (5) measurement of progress. Examples from treatment of disordered children are included throughout the chapter.

Before discussing phonological remediation in detail, it is important to review certain principles that we consider basic, regardless of the approach adopted. These principles are important because they determine the manner in which remediation is planned and implemented. The principles include:

1. Developing a treatment plan based on all underlying factors that may contribute to the etiology of the disorder
2. Considering each child as an individual
3. Using normal acquisition data as a guide for planning treatment
4. Using a comprehensive framework of phonology for planning treatment
5. Teaching children to monitor responses
6. Systematically measuring progress

Each of these principles is discussed below and referred to later in the chapter.

The first principle refers to developing a treatment plan based on all factors that may relate to the phonological disorder. Such factors include: (1) auditory abilities; (2) structural adequacy; (3) motoric abilities necessary to plan and execute sound patterns and suprasegmental features of speech; (4) linguistic knowledge, especially phonological knowledge; (5) cognitive abilities; and (6) psychosocial considerations. As seen in Chapter 5, the etiology of many severe phonological disorders cannot be determined. Therefore it is critical to consider all possible factors that may influence the development of a sound system. Unfortunately, remediation approaches tend to focus on one aspect of the problem and overlook others. For example, many approaches are based on development of motoric skills, to the exclusion of possible linguistic problems. More recently, it has been recognized that some disordered children have little difficulty with motoric production but cannot systematically use the sounds they can produce. As a result, current treatment approaches attempt to establish phonological concepts (e.g., contrasts between sounds) but do not attempt to establish motoric skills as well. This "either/or" approach to treatment can result in limited effectiveness. The alternative to basing remediation on a few factors is to conduct a broad-based evaluation including the factors listed above and then integrating the results into a comprehensive treatment plan for each child.

The second principle, considering each child as an individual, is a corollary of the first. It calls attention to the individual differences described in earlier chapters for both normal and disordered children. Each child has a unique history and constellation of skills that must be considered when planning and implementing a treatment program.

In the third principle, use of normal acquisition data is recommended as one guideline for planning treatment. As seen in Chapter 2, a child must master the sounds and syllable structure of the system, eliminate phonological processes, and use phonemic contrasts among other skills. Data are now available that indicate how a child acquires some aspects of the system most naturally. For example, some sounds emerge first in word-final position and then are gradually used in other word positions. Treatment may progress most efficiently if goals are selected that follow natural sequences of development. Normal acquisition data can be applied and evaluated systematically to determine how this principle is most effective.

The fourth principle is the use of a comprehensive framework of phonology for planning treatment. Otherwise, treatment tends to be directed toward one aspect of acquisition, e.g., mastery of a sound inventory or elimination of phonological processes. These two approaches represent only part of the phonological system. Recent data about phonological acquisition reveal that children must master a variety of skills; and these skills should be incorporated into treatment to facilitate acquisition of the adult system with maximum efficiency.

Teaching children to monitor responses is the fifth principle. This principle is based on the notion that children should be actively involved not only in perceiving and producing speech patterns but in judging the accuracy of the responses as well. This involvement forces the child to be aware of responses and to recognize his or her own role in changes that can be made. Without such involvement, it is possible for the child to respond automatically, without incorporating the new behaviors into his or her linguistic system.

The last principle, which was identified as the final objective of assessment in Chapter 6, specifies that progress should be systematically measured. Measurement includes at least three basic components: (1) initial testing to determine entry-level skills at the beginning of treatment; (2) testing to determine if there is improvement in what is being taught; and (3) testing to determine if there is generalization to material that has not been taught. Without the measurement of progress and generalization, there is no way to evaluate the effectiveness of a treatment program. In addition, there is no way to ensure that the child is incorporating a new skill into his or her system. At the present time it is difficult to tell which factors contribute to success or failure of a treatment approach.

The principles described above are not intended to encompass every possible consideration that should be made about phonological remediation, but they do reflect ideas we consider basic to any treatment approach. The knowledge and beliefs that one brings to treatment determine the course of remediation. Therefore it is important that each person actively develop principles that guide phonological remediation. With this perspective as our basis for remediation, application of phonological concepts to treatment of disordered phonology is described.

Phonological Remediation

It is important to clarify what is meant by *phonological* remediation. To characterize it concisely, it: (1) is based on the systematic nature of phonology; (2) is characterized by conceptual, rather than motoric, activities; and (3) has generalization as its ultimate goal.

Phonological remediation emphasizes the systematic nature of sound patterns in child speech. Rather than viewing sound segments as isolated units, they are considered in relation to: (1) how they are used contrastively; and (2) how they are combined in different word structures. These functions, or roles, for sound segments in the linguistic system are often apparent through patterns that affect groups of sounds that are similar in place, manner, or voicing features. In other words, the patterns often involve natural sound classes, (e.g., substitution of stops for fricatives) or word structures (e.g., final consonant deletion). Treatment is directed toward a sound class (e.g., acquisition of the *class* of fricatives, instead of one fricative at a time) or toward a word structure (e.g., including consonants in word-final position).

When a phonological approach to remediation is used, a child's phonological system is usually described using one of two basic frameworks: *distinctive features* or *phonological processes*. When a distinctive feature framework is used, features are described as being present and absent in a child's system; the underlying treatment goal is to teach the absent feature. When a phonological process framework is used, substitutions or word structure changes involving classes of sounds are identified; the treatment goal is to eliminate the occurrence of the process. Each framework accounts for substitution errors in a similar way. For example, a child may use [t] for /k/, [d] for /g/, and [n] for /ŋ/. In a distinctive feature framework the error pattern would be described this way: [+ velar] sounds become [+ alveolar]. In a phonological process framework the implication is that the class of velars has been changed to alveolars; the pattern would be referred to as the process of Velar Fronting. Thus the same surface speech pattern can be described using a distinctive feature or a phonological process framework.

However, treatment that incorporates the process framework extends beyond the traditional feature framework because patterns of Final Consonant Deletion, Cluster Reduction, and Assimilation are also considered. The concepts of features and processes are not usually considered in relation to each other.

Another characteristic of phonological remediation is its *conceptual* nature (Blache et al., 1981; Fokes, 1982; Weiner, 1981b). This characterization comes from the linguistic units (e.g., contrasts, features, and phonological processes) that are the basis of training. Although these units are abstract concepts that cannot be directly observed, surface speech patterns can be seen. These surface patterns lead to the assumption that a child lacks underlying cognitive knowledge, particularly that sounds contrast meaning. Unfortunately, activities are often planned without testing this assumption.

Conceptually based treatment activities are designed to provide meaningful communication situations. In a typical activity, the child is presented with contrastive minimal word pairs and is required to produce the target sound correctly. There is a communication breakdown if the child fails to produce the sound that distinguishes the words; for example, the target sound /s/ is contrasted with /t/ in the pair *sip–tip*. If the child substitutes [t] for /s/, listener uncertainty is created. The uncertainty results in a communication breakdown, which supposedly forces the child to become aware of the error and change an underlying concept. It is not clear, however, whether the child's *improvement* in production is due to a cognitive restructuring of a concept or to the production practice and feedback that are also part of the activity. Perhaps it is a combination of cognitive and production factors. The notion of *conceptual* treatment is rather vague at this point and needs further empirical study.

Finally, if phonological remediation is successful, *generalization* should occur. Generalization has been defined as the ability to produce untrained phonemes or words that have the target feature or phoneme. For example, once a [+strident] phoneme such as /s/ has been learned, other strident phonemes such as /f/ or /ʃ/ are tested to determine if they are correctly produced as well. The underlying premise is that there will be correct production of the other phonemes in the class because they have the place, manner, or voicing feature that the child has learned.

This definition is narrow, because generalization also implies correct production of untrained linguistic units at the conversational level in situations outside the training setting. Few studies have addressed the broader concept of generalization. Nonetheless, it is an important therapeutic concept; if correct production of untrained sounds can be obtained, the amount of time in treatment is reduced. Although generalization is considered an important result of phonological remediation, most empirical studies have reported limited success. After a discussion of phonological remediation studies, generalization is reviewed in more detail and suggestions made about ways to achieve optimal generalization.

In summary, phonological remediation has been characterized as *systematic* because sound classes are usually the target for remediation. Treatment activities are *conceptual* in nature, because they focus on abstract units, e.g., features, phonological processes, or contrasts. The activities tend to require meaningful communication, with little emphasis on motoric practice. When treatment is completed, *generalization* of the target feature or concept to untrained sounds or words is tested. With this description of phonological remediation as background, the application of distinctive features and phonological processes to treatment is discussed. Information about these two approaches comes primarily from empirical studies. In addition, a treatment approach based on the elimination of phonological processes (Hodson and Paden, 1983) is described.

Application of Distinctive Features to Phonological Remediation

Remediation based on distinctive features was most popular during the 1970s (Costello and Onstine, 1976; McReynolds and Bennett, 1972; McReynolds and Engmann, 1975; Weiner and Bankson, 1978), although there continues to be interest in using this framework for treatment (Blache et al., 1981; Ruder and Bunce, 1981). Distinctive features have been considered basic units that provide the linguistic contrasts essential to the acquisition of phonemes and phone classes (McReynolds and Bennett, 1972). Thus features function to distinguish two phonemes or one sound class from another. The goal of distinctive feature programs was to establish production of a sound class by teaching a feature as it occurred in a sound. It was assumed that generalization to other members of the sound class would occur spontaneously. Features that were totally or partially absent from the child's repertoire were identified by lengthy analysis procedures.

The features were taught using activities that contrasted phonemes that differed in the presence or absence of a feature. For example, when teaching the feature [+velar], /k/ would be used to represent the target feature and it would be contrasted with a [-velar] phoneme, e.g., /t/. The contrasting phoneme was usually the one that was substituted for the target phoneme. This teaching strategy implicitly suggested that a child learns a *contrast* between features. Within this contrastive framework, activities differed from program to program. They varied from traditional production drills in which the sound and its substitution were practiced motorically to production of minimal word pairs in communication situations that emphasized the necessity of distinguishing among the words. The linguistic stimuli were usually words; sometimes a traditional teaching hierarchy was followed, beginning with syllables and progressing through a series of linguistic levels to conversational speech. In some of the studies, auditory discrimination tasks were included. At the end of treatment, generalization of the feature was measured.

There are three major contributions that evolved from the distinctive feature treatment programs. First, selection of target phonemes was based on a sound class as opposed to isolated phonemes. The concept of features emphasizes the phonological characteristics that phonemes have in common and aids the clinician in teaching the "critical elements" common to several phonemes. As a result of learning a feature, disordered children may acquire a class of sounds that has a common feature, e.g., velars, rather than acquiring the velar sounds one by one.

Viewing generalization as a goal of treatment is a second contribution of the distinctive framework to treatment. When generalization (e.g., correct production) to untrained sounds is measured, the sound system is viewed in a more integrated way because the clinician determines how treatment has affected a class of sounds, as opposed to single sounds. Thus treatment is based on changing the phonological system and not just on teaching a child to produce sounds.

The third contribution is the use of contrasts in teaching. This teaching technique, whether it is motoric or conceptual, may enable the child to isolate more easily the critical elements to be learned. The distinctive feature approach has demonstrated the value of allowing the child to become cognitively aware of the units he was learning. Although the ideas of manner, place, and voicing features and contrastive teaching are not new, the work with distinctive features served to integrate phonological concepts with more traditional treatment techniques.

The application of distinctive features to treatment has limitations. The most serious limitation lies in the feature systems that are adopted as the basis for treatment. A variety of systems has been used, as described in Chapter 1. Because these systems are intended to describe abstract phonemes and not the actual physical gestures of speech (Parker, 1976; Walsh, 1974), they were not entirely satisfactory for describing some of the productions in child speech. For example, whereas the *features* for voiced and voiceless stops are the same in initial and final position, the *physical gestures* are not the same owing to differences in aspiration, voice onset time, and vowel transition characteristics. Because there is not a one-to-one relationship between productions required in the two word positions, Parker (1976) suggested that there is probably no generalization from initial to final position. This example illustrates the necessity to consider motoric implementation of abstract features when using a distinctive approach in remediation.

An additional problem of feature systems is the lack of agreement about how to distinguish among sounds. For example, the noisy, turbulent feature of the fricative /s/ is described as [+ sibilant] (Singh and Polen, 1972), [+ strident] (Chomsky and Halle, 1968), and as having the feature of "constricted closure" (Irwin and Wong, 1983). It is not clear which system of features is most appropriate for describing normal or disordered child phonology. However, because the system determines what is taught in therapy, it should adequately describe the nature of the speech signal as it occurs in child speech. We have adopted a system of articulatory features in this book that we have found useful in describing phonological systems that are developing.

Another limitation of teaching distinctive features is reflected in the results of generalization testing. In treatment studies, responses for some untrained phonemes were more accurate after training whereas other phonemes were not more accurate. The success or failure in obtaining generalization may be due either to selecting *features* as the target of treatment or to the *approach* used to teach the features. It is possible that the treatment procedures themselves have limited the amount of generalization. All of these limitations lead to a diminishing interest in trying to teach features and attention shifted toward phonological processes as an alternative.

Application of Phonological Processes to Phonological Remediation

A phonological process has been described as a systematic simplification of adult words, usually through change of a sound class or a word structure. Several people have provided descriptions of treatment procedures that incorporate a phonological process framework (Edwards, 1980a; Elbert et al., 1980; Ferrier and Davis, 1973; Hodson and Paden, 1983; Ingram, 1976; Weiner, 1979). The procedures include: (1) selection of processes to eliminate; (2) the order in which to eliminate processes; and (3) treatment techniques. The suggested techniques include practice of the consonant in words or activities that require the child to contrast the correct and incorrect productions. As mentioned for distinctive features earlier, the training procedures for eliminating processes do not differ greatly from traditional approaches. However, suggestions for selection of treatment goals are innovative. Classes of sounds (e.g., fricatives) and word structures (e.g., word-final position) are the focus of change. The processes suggested for elimination were those that: (1) contribute greatly to poor intelligibility (Edwards, 1980a; Weiner, 1979); (2) establish sounds in a variety of sound classes and word structures; (3) are eliminated early in the course of normal acquisition (Weiner, 1979); (4) typically persist in children with disordered phonology (Edwards, 1980a); or (5) occur more than 40% of the time in the child's speech (Hodson and Paden, 1983). Typically, more than one sound is trained for each process. Generalization of trained responses to untrained consonants is a primary goal of eliminating processes, just as it is in distinctive feature remediation.

Although these ideas about eliminating processes are valuable because they provide new options for treatment, they must be viewed with caution. They are only suggestions, not reports of treatment studies. At present, there are two empirical studies in the literature using phonological processes in treatment (McReynolds and Elbert, 1981; Weiner, 1981b). The processes, linguistic level trained, and the training technique that was used for each study are presented in Table 7.1.

The training techniques were very different: McReynolds and

Table 7.1 Characteristics of Two Treatment Studies

Study	Processes	Linguistic level trained	Training technique
McReynolds and Elbert (1981)	Cluster Reduction (s,r,l clusters)	Nonsense syllables	Imitative nonsense drill
Weiner (1981b)	Final C Deletion Stopping Cluster Reduction	Words	Contrast of minimal pair words

Elbert trained one exemplar of a process (e.g., /st-/ to eliminate Cluster Reduction), whereas Weiner trained two to four exemplars for each process, e.g., fricatives /f,v,s,z/ to eliminate Stopping. The clusters were trained in imitative nonsense drills, whereas the processes in Weiner's study were presented in meaningful activities that required accurate production of minimal pair words. These differences indicate that there is not just one approach for phonological process treatment. Instead, the factor common to all process treatment is the underlying organizational concept of a process, i.e., changes affecting a sound class or word structure.

Successful generalization would support the notion of an underlying process. Weiner reported successful generalization to sounds and words that were not practiced, for all three processes. In the McReynolds and Elbert study, there was generalization for *within-class* clusters, e.g., /st-/ training generalized to other /s/ clusters. However, only one of six children had *across-class* generalization, e.g., generalization from /s/ clusters to /r/ clusters. Based on these results, McReynolds and Elbert suggested that "misarticulating children may not always be using simplifications which are based on application of general phonological processes. The errors tend, instead, to be production errors on specific sounds." Along the same lines, they stated that patterns of errors "do not always reflect processes."

The reservations that McReynolds and Elbert had about underlying processes are important, because it is possible that all children do not organize and simplify all productions according to processes. DE, the first child described in Chapter 6, may be such a child. However, there are other factors that may account for the limited across-class generalization. First, processes may affect or represent sound classes in a different way than word structures. Therefore learning a feature of sounds (e.g., [+strident]) may be different from learning the structure of words, e.g., consonant clusters. Second, it is not surprising that training one exemplar of an /s/ cluster (e.g., /st-/) resulted in no generalization to an /r/ cluster. Generalization from /s/ to /r/ would not be expected because the features of these two sounds are so different. Third, the training itself may have limited the generalization, because it was nonmeaningful and imitative. Optimal generalization may occur when sounds to be incorporated into the linguistic system are used meaningfully. Finally, no mention was made of the children's ability to produce /s,r,l/ as singletons before treatment began. Generalization is unlikely to occur if a motoric production is not possible.

These factors, which possibly limit generalization, are raised to illustrate how much we have to learn about treatment based on the concept of phonological processes. Carefully designed studies such as that of McReynolds and Elbert are essential to the better understanding of phonological treatment procedures.

Phonological Approach to Remediation

Hodson and Paden (1983) described an alternative approach for eliminating phonological processes in unintelligible children. The approach is eclectic in nature because it combines the application of phonological concepts with more traditional training procedures. It is described briefly here; the reader is referred to Hodson and Paden (1983) for a more detailed description of the approach.

Hodson and Paden presented five underlying concepts that serve as the basis for their approach:

1. Phonological acquisition is a gradual process.
2. Children with normal hearing typically acquire the adult sound system primarily by listening.
3. As the child acquires new speech patterns, he associates kinesthetic with auditory sensations, which enables later self-monitoring.
4. Phonetic environment can facilitate correct sound production.
5. Children tend to generalize new articulation skills to other targets. (pp. 44–49)

These concepts emphasize the use of information about normal acquisition to select intervention goals and plan treatment procedures. In addition, the concepts support the premise that children learn the phonological system with sound classes and word structures as basic organizational constructs (hence supporting the notion that generalization can occur within classes or structures).

Acquisition of "new sound patterns" is the goal of the treatment approach; this goal is achieved by first identifying the phonological processes that occur in more than 40% of the possible contexts on the Assessment of Phonological Processes (Hodson, 1980). The cutoff of 40% is suggested because results of clinical work using this approach indicate that processes that occur in fewer than 40% of the words tested are spontaneously reduced without treatment. An average of three to six processes are selected for remediation; the purpose of selecting several processes is to provide broad-based stimulation of the sound system in a very short period of time. A minimum of two target phonemes is typically selected for remediation of each process.

Table 7.2 Patterns and Initial and Final Phonemes Representing Two Treatment Cycles for Two Children

Child 1	Child 2
Cycle 1	**Cycle 1**
Prevocalic velars	Postvocalic velars
/k/[Ia]	/k/[F]
Stridency	Stridency
/sp/[I]	/ps/[F]
/st/[I]	/ts/[F]
/f/[I]	/sk/[I]
Liquids	/sp/[I]
/l/[I]	Liquids
/r/[I]	/r/[I]
Cycle 2	**Cycle 2**
Prevocalic velars	Stridency
/k/[I], /g/[I]	Plurals
Stridency	/sk/, /sp/[I]
/sp/, /st/[I]	/st/[I]
/sm/[I]	/sm/, /sn/[I]
/sn/[I]	It's a non-/s/[I]
/sk/[I]	It's a /s/[I]
It's a non-/s/[Ib]	/s/[I]
It's a /s/[I]	/f/[I]
/tʃ/[F]	/t/[I]
/f/[F]	Liquids
/f/[I]	/l/[I]
Liquids	/r/ clusters
/l/[I]	
/r/[I]	

Adapted from Hodson and Paden (1983). I = initial phonemes; F = final phonemes.

[a]Each line on which phoneme(s) are presented represents 1 week of training.

[b]The phrase "It's a _____" was used first without and then with /s/ words in order to develop the ability to produce two stridents in the same utterance.

Table 7.2 summarizes treatment goals for two children seen by Hodson and Paden. The patterns to be learned and the phonemes selected for each pattern are listed. For example, for the first child, initial /sp/ and /st/ clusters and /f/ singleton were selected to target stridency, whereas four strident clusters were selected for the second child. Each process is worked on for a minimum of two sessions. Therefore the phonemes are not trained until the child reaches a certain criterion level of accuracy (e.g.,

90%) but are stimulated intensely for only a few sessions. Stimulating five or six patterns usually takes a period of 6–12 weeks. Hodson and Paden referred to the period as a "cycle" because the same processes are worked on again in subsequent training periods or are "re-cycled" until they are substantially reduced in frequency of occurrence. They stated that generalization may not be apparent during the first period of training but begins to occur steadily in subsequent training cycles. Dismissal from treatment is reported for most children after two or three cycles of treatment.

It is important to note the difference in the two children's treatment goals presented in Table 7.2. Although there are certain similarities, e.g., the patterns targeted in cycle 1, the phonemes selected for each pattern differ. As Hodson and Paden (1983) clearly pointed out, "There is no 'cook book' order for selecting targets, since the clients' requirements and capabilities will differ, even when the same deficient pattern is shared." Based on our own clinical work with Hodson and Paden's approach, we concur that each child has individual needs when formulating cycles. Therefore the cycles in Table 7.2 are illustrative only of potential cycles.

At the beginning and end of each treatment session, Hodson and Paden employed a listening technique called *auditory bombardment*. With the child wearing an auditory trainer, a machine that amplifies auditory input, the trainer is set at a comfortable loudness level, and the child listens to the clinician read a list of approximately 20 words containing the target phoneme. No response is required; the child sits and listens for about 2 minutes while engaging in some quiet hand activity. According to Hodson and Paden, the purpose of the bombardment is to help develop "auditory images," so that the child will be able to monitor incorrect productions. For the rest of the treatment session, the target sounds are practiced in words during play activities in order to build kinesthetic images. When necessary, tactile cues or minimal pair contrasts are used to establish the production of a sound.

Hodson and Paden's approach has appeal because it offers innovative ideas for remediation. The aspect that is most promising is the notion of cycles based on the stimulation of several sound classes for short periods. When mastering the phonological system, a normal child works toward gradual yet simultaneous mastery of several phonemes from different sound classes. Hodson and Paden's approach resembles the normal acquisition process by providing practice with several phonemes, thus stimulating the child's system to change but allowing it to do so at the child's own rate. This aspect of Hodson and Paden's approach merits empirical investigation, especially to determine if teaching in cycles is appropriate for all phonologically disordered children.

Hodson and Paden (1983) reported that over a 6-year period they worked with 125 unintelligible children, ages 3–9 years. They were able to dismiss the children from therapy as intelligible within 18 months or less. It is not clear whether the success that they report is due to using a phonological process framework or to a combination of other variables. Some of the variables that could be isolated for study include:

1. Target selection based on a cutoff score of 40% occurrence of a process
2. Cyclic training based on stimulation of several target sounds for short periods
3. Auditory bombardment of target sounds.

In their description of this approach, Hodson and Paden did not document the course of progress, nor did they conduct an experimental study of the variables. Such a unique approach to remediation deserves and demands empirical verification. It is hoped that future research in phonological remediation will investigate variables from Hodson and Paden's approach.

Critique of Phonological Remediation There are some similarities between remediation based on phonological processes and distinctive features. Both frameworks offer a systematic way to describe speech patterns. However, processes provide a broader framework than features because they incorporate word structure patterns as well as sound substitution. In addition, processes can be compared to normal acquisition patterns for guidance about what to select for treatment. Activities that incorporate the use of meaningful communication as the basis for change (common to both distinctive feature and process remediation) are an important alternative to exclusive use of production drill.

The last point raises a limitation regarding phonologically based treatment, i.e., the child's need to learn how to *produce* a sound. A basic level of motoric ability is an essential prerequisite for success with conceptual treatment tasks. However, this issue is not often addressed in discussions of phonological remediation. In conclusion, treatment based on a phonological framework is virtually untested. At present, distinctive features and phonological processes are most useful in providing a systematic way to describe sound patterns that may be used in the selection of treatment goals and in measuring treatment progress.

Generalization

As described earlier, a basic goal of phonological remediation is generalization of the trained feature or segment to untrained linguistic units. Studies assessing generalization have only considered correct production in untrained sounds and words. Generalization results have been equivocal at best (Costello and Onstine, 1976; McReynolds and Bennett, 1972; McReynolds and Elbert, 1981); that is, some generalization occurred across a sound class, but all sounds were not mastered. As shown in Chapter 2, normal children do not acquire features across a sound class but seem to acquire them individually within segments. However, Ingram (1976) suggested that generalization might be a reasonable goal in a clinical setting if certain variables are controlled during treatment. Some of the more important variables to consider include:

1. Number of target phonemes that represent the feature
2. Variety of feature combinations among the trained phonemes
3. Ability to produce the sounds prior to training
4. Characteristics of individual children

Two primary reasons for a lack of generalization to untrained linguistic units are that: (1) not enough sounds are trained that represent the feature; and (2) the trained and untrained sounds do not have enough features in common. As an example of these points, the generalization results of a study by McReynolds and Bennett (1972) are presented. The feature *stridency* was taught using /f/ as the target sound, and generalization was measured to four other strident sounds. Training was conducted at the syllable level; generalization was measured at the word level. The amount of improvement for the sounds was as follows: [s] 100%, [z] 60%, [v] 47%, and [tʃ] 94%.

The major articulatory features of /f/ are [-voice] and [-labial], as well as stridency. When considering the features of the untrained phonemes, there were a variety of differences from /f/: /s/ differed from /f/ in a place feature, /v/ differed in voicing, /z/ differed in both place and voicing, and /tʃ/ differed in place and manner. Therefore each test sound had other features that combined with stridency. Training two exemplars simultaneously (e.g., /f/ and /z/) would have presented more varied features (voiced and voiceless, labial and alveolar) to show that stridency can be combined with a variety of features. It is unlikely that a child can establish the concept of a sound class without enough varied examples to represent the category. Costello and Onstine (1976) used this notion of multiple exemplars when they trained /θ/ and /s/ for the feature [+ continuant]. Generalization was measured to /ð,z,ʃ/. The accuracy of performance on the training and generalization sounds was typically above 80%, but there were scores below 80% for [ð] and [ʃ]. These results suggest that teaching multiple exemplars may increase the likelihood of generalization but may not be sufficient for optimal generalization.

Another reason for limited generalization may be a lack of motoric ability. If a child cannot produce a sound, e.g., [tʃ], it is not likely that training on another sound, e.g., [f], will result in correct production. It is important to determine if a child can produce a sound before beginning treatment. If there are sounds that cannot be produced in a class of sounds, some motoric training should precede any sort of conceptual training. Elbert and McReynolds (1978) showed that generalization occurred more rapidly once a child could imitate a sound.

Yet another explanation for limited generalization is the characteristics of individual children. The process of generalization may be "highly variable across individuals" (Bernthal and Bankson, 1981). Some children may easily recognize features that are common to several sounds, generalizing production from one sound to many. Other children may not be able to do this, especially those with language disorders that involve other components of the language system. Children with limited motoric ability may also have difficulty generalizing to untrained sounds. Finally, each child has a unique constellation of errors; different error patterns may result in different generalization results. Studies that have considered generalization have not attempted to determine if the child has good potential for generalization. The variables mentioned above merit consideration empirically in order to allow predictions about prognosis and how to select treatment goals.

In conclusion, generalization is a desirable goal of phonological remediation. However, it does not happen automatically with all children. In a report on the technology of generalization, Stokes and Baer (1977) stated that "the best course of action seems to be that of systematic measurement and analysis of variables" that may have resulted in generalization. They offered a variety of ways to achieve successful generalization to new settings, people, and more complex linguistic levels. One important way was to use systematic probes to identify where generalization does and does not occur, so that the training program can be modified to facilitate generalization. They suggested establishing natural contingencies, e.g., parental, teacher, and peer support, that maintain correct production so that contrived reinforcement is not necessary. They also suggested informing the client about the need for generalization through the use of self-monitoring techniques. These suggestions imply a broader view of generalization than has been described in the literature in phonological remediation. This view should be incorporated systematically into clinical treatment and research of phonological disorders.

Summary In the preceding sections, the application of distinctive features and phonological processes to treatment has been reviewed, particularly in relation to generalization, which is a basic goal of phonological remediation. The greatest contributions of the phonological framework have been in target selection and measurement of progress.

Treatment Variables

There are several variables in addition to generalization that require careful attention in treatment. In this section of the chapter, variables related to the planning and implementation of treatment are discussed. These variables, which reflect ideas and concerns that have recently appeared in the literature, are explored in five major categories: (1) linguistic content; (2) structure of remediation sessions; (3) remediation techniques; (4) definition of a correct response and criteria for sound mastery; and (5) measurement of progress.

Linguistic Content

An important issue is selection of the phonological unit that is the focus in treatment and how the phonological goals relate to the rest of the linguistic system. When selecting treatment targets, *distinctive features* or *phonological processes* are often the focus. However, because these concepts are abstract in nature, words that represent the underlying unit are selected as the training unit. Isolated sounds or syllables become the target only when a child has motoric difficulty producing the target sound in words. Therefore in phonological remediation, treatment is directed toward establishing features, contrasts, or sound classes in words. Little empirical attention has been paid recently to establishing the words in more complex linguistic structures; apparently it is assumed that this will happen automatically.

Traditionally, target selection has been guided by normative data for single sounds (Templin, 1957). Information about normal acquisition has now shown that there are developmental factors to consider in addition to the ages of mastery for single sounds. There is information about the systematic way that children acquire sound classes and word structures, as well as how and when they eliminate phonological processes. This knowledge can be used to aid in selecting remediation targets. For example, we now realize that sounds from all classes begin to *emerge* very early. According to Ingram (1981, p. 98), the following repertoire of sounds in initial and final position is typical for normal 2-year-old children:

Initial	Final
m n	m n
b p d t g k	p t k
f s h	
w	

In addition, clusters begin emerging at around 2 years of age (Greenlee, 1974). Therefore although certain phonemes (e.g., fricatives, affricates, or liquids) or sound combinations (e.g., clusters) are *mastered* later, they *emerge* very early. If one uses normal acquisition information as a guide, early treatment goals would include phonemes from these classes, as well as clusters, in order to facilitate emergence. Hodson and Paden (1983) followed this approach in the selection of processes to eliminate by stimulating the emergence of phonemes from a variety of sound classes. Treatment that encourages *emergence* of phonemes and provides practice across the whole system without requiring mastery approximates normal acquisition. Such an approach may provide the most beneficial stimulation for a child's overall development.

Recent normal acquisition data may also be used in relation to phoneme position in the word. Traditionally, phonemes are taught first in word-initial position. However, as shown in Chapter 2, it seems that fricatives and velars may emerge first in final position in normal children. This pattern of emergence has not been documented in disordered children; however, observations of disordered children in treatment indicate that velars and fricatives first emerge spontaneously or are most easily stimulated in final position for some children. Such information is important because it offers alternatives to goal selection that may facilitate more rapid progress. If a child is more easily stimulated to produce a sound in a certain word position, less time should be required to establish it initially and then it possibly would generalize to other word positions more rapidly.

These examples are only two ways that information from normal acquisition can be used to select targets for treatment. There is still much that is not known about the acquisition of the phonological system; as new information becomes available, it should be considered and used when making decisions about treatment. Only through such application will we know which aspects of normal acquisition are applicable to the disordered population.

In the meantime, a question arises about how to use traditional single-sound normative information in relation to newer information. In terms of selecting a sound such as a fricative or a cluster to teach as an early target, one could use Sander's (1972) normative information as a guide to select a fricative that emerges early, e.g., /f/ or /s/. This selection is compatible with information about early sound emergence. In addition, one should probe to determine if the sound can be produced; if it cannot be, it is not a good choice for training. In short, the clinician must be able to creatively combine information about normal acquisition from a variety of sources and apply it to each child's unique error patterns and skills.

In addition to using information from normal acquisition to select treatment goals, the characteristics of disordered phonology should be used as well. It is possible that the sequence of normal acquisition will not be applicable for many disordered children (Dunn and Till, 1982), especially those with an auditory, structural, or neuromotor disability. There are characteristics to consider about disordered phonology in addition to the use of distinctive features and phonological processes. As discussed in Chapter 5, some of these characteristics include Sound Preference (substitution of one phoneme for many others), restricted use of the sound inventory, or use of unusual processes, e.g., Backing and Glottal Replacement. These are only a few behaviors that could serve as input for treatment goals.

Another consideration for linguistic content is the relationship between the phonological system and the other components of the linguistic system. Children with phonological problems are often described as having other linguistic problems as well, particularly syntactic problems (Panagos, 1978). Suggestions have been made to formulate treatment goals that simultaneously consider phonology and syntax, semantic relations, or the lexicon (Dunn and Barron, 1982; Schwartz et al., 1980). However, there has been very little empirical study of simultaneous remediation of various components of the linguistic system. Matheny and Panagos (1978) taught either syntax or phonology in two groups of 8 children who were 5 and 6 years old. All of the children were disordered in both linguistic components. Both groups made significant improvement in both components regardless of the training received. The authors concluded that "manipulations of a child's linguistic system at any level (such as sounds, syllables, phrases, and sentences) are likely to produce broader linguistic results than anticipated." Improvement in more than one linguistic component, regardless of what is taught, implies that simultaneous teaching of different components may not be necessary. However, these results were based on very structured training procedures, so it is not clear how much one can generalize these results to other types of treatment or other children.

Until more empirical work has been done, certain guidelines can be followed for coordinating phonology goals with other linguistic components. When planning phonological goals: (1) words chosen for training should be within the child's vocabulary; and (2) sentence patterns should be within syntactic–semantic abilities. In teaching syntactic–semantic skills, the lexicon selected should be within the child's phonological capabilities in terms of both the sounds and the syllable structure of the words. For example, when teaching sentence patterns with *contraction* as the target, the clinician should probe to see if the child is capable of producing the final clusters in the target words (e.g., can't, don't). If the child cannot produce the cluster, the phonological constraint could increase the complexity of the task. Finally, if there is simultaneous training of different components, e.g., phonology and a particular semantic relation (e.g., action–object), words being trained phonologically could be incorporated into practice with the semantic relation once they are accurately produced in the phonological task. These suggestions avoid the separation of linguistic training into isolated components, which is an artificial dichotomy that does not exist in natural language use.

Structure of Remediation Sessions

During the late 1960s and early 1970s, operant conditioning procedures provided the major framework for phonological remediation (Costello, 1977; Costello and Onstine, 1976; Mowrer, 1977). The structure of treatment sessions centered around programmed instruction, including concepts of antecedent events, responses, and consequences. The guidelines provided by programmed instruction were useful in helping a clinician identify systematic steps to follow in achieving specific behaviors. A goal of this highly structured programming was to provide as much practice (i.e., as many responses) as possible during a treatment session. This goal resulted in drill-oriented sessions, which deemphasized conceptual decision-making on the client's part. In addition, sessions that incorporated operant techniques provided little opportunity for natural communication between the clinician and the client. During recent years, as language acquisition research has emphasized the importance of natural interactions, the structure of phonological remediation sessions has changed. Therapy sessions are more likely to incorporate communication-oriented activities, which give the client the opportunity to use the phonological targets in meaningful ways.

One type of less structured approach, referred to as Theraplay, was described by Kupperman et al. (1980). The approach was based on parent–child interaction patterns; the children and clinicians interacted in a series of activities including babbling, singing songs, counting, playing peek-a-boo, talking, and so on. The child's target phonemes were identified as part of the play activities. However, sound production was never taught, no direct responses were required of the children, and no correction of the child's speech was provided. Six children (ages 3;2–6;6) with delayed phonology participated in the study. There were 10–12 treatment sessions for each child. The authors concluded that the method was successful because there was an average reduction of 10.8 errors on the articulation test administered at the beginning and end of treatment. This improvement was achieved after only 6 weeks of treatment. The authors suggested that the children tended to be systematic in their improvement; for example, one child began to include final consonants, and another began producing clusters. The authors were justifiably cautious in their interpretation of the results because many contaminating variables were not controlled. In addition, a single-word articulation test is a limited tool for measuring progress.

Nevertheless, this description of Theraplay is presented to show that: (1) progress can be achieved through interactive communicative situations; and (2) motoric drill is not necessarily a requirement for progress. However, interactive treatment sessions imply the need for very careful planning, so that a child systematically hears and practices the target units. In the Theraplay approach, the clinician controlled the play and provided rich, systematic stimulation of the target phoneme. In some ways Theraplay is similar to Hodson and Paden's (1983) approach because it provides broad-based stimulation in an interactive, game-like setting. For some children, especially those with good motoric and linguistic ability, the interactive approach may be a viable alternative to more structured treatment sessions. This type of structure could be studied empirically in order to determine which children are more likely to benefit from interactive structure.

Shriberg and Kwiatkowski (1982b) designed a series of three studies with just these concerns about treatment structure. They had found in their treatment work with younger children that "the efficient stimulus–response paradigms of behaviorism were not effective. These children did not like to 'drill,' no matter what the pay-off." In order to study the effectiveness (measured by the number of correct responses) and efficiency (measured by the number of responses per session) of various types of treatment structure, they developed four management modes that were used to teach a variety of phonological structures. The modes included:

(1) *drill*—a highly structured and efficient stimulus-response mode,
(2) *drill play*—similar to drill, except that a motivational event that was fun for the child was included,
(3) *structured play*—the training stimuli were presented as part of play activities; feedback about incorrect responses was optional, and
(4) *play*—stimulus and response events occurred as natural components of play activities. (Shriberg and Kwiatkowski, 1982b, pp. 246–247)

Shriberg and Kwiatkowski concluded that drill and drill play were significantly more effective and efficient than structured play or play. They were unsuccessful in identifying a subgroup of children who performed better in one mode than another. The clinicians who carried out the training for the study preferred all modes but drill; however, the consensus was that the match between the child and the structural mode was the most important factor to consider. The authors concluded that "clear-cut guidelines for the selection of an appropriate management structure for individual children have not emerged from these studies." They emphasized the need to consider the child's personality as well as the target response to be learned and the stage of remediation when planning for a structural mode.

In summary, there is a trend in phonological remediation away from highly structured treatment sessions characterized by the operant conditioning paradigm toward more interactive, communication-based sessions. This trend is valuable in that it allows the clinician and the child more freedom to interact meaningfully about the linguistic content that is being learned. However, it is important not to abandon the rigor that operant conditioning techniques provided, especially the careful analysis and sequencing of behaviors to be acquired and the systematic measurement of progress. Ideally, there will be a balance in planning remediation using various types of treatment structure as they apply to individual children in various stages of remediation. Attention to the abilities and constellation of errors of individual children is an essential part of any remediation planning.

Remediation Techniques

The next section on treatment variables addresses techniques for presenting the content of a treatment session. Techniques include auditory training and self-monitoring as well as use of facilitating contexts. The reader is referred to Bernthal and Bankson (1981) for a review of other techniques, especially establishment and maintenance of new phonological behaviors.

Auditory Training and Self-Monitoring Auditory training tasks are frequently part of phonological remediation. The tasks have taken many forms, including identification of target phonemes, discrimination between target and substitute phonemes, and bombardment of target phonemes. In spite of the long-term interest in training auditory perceptual skills (Powers, 1971; Van Riper, 1972; Winitz, 1975), there has been little empirical investigation of this topic as it relates to remediation. Most attention has been given to auditory discrimination training.

There is a longstanding assumption that a child must be able to discriminate the error phoneme from a target phoneme before production training can begin (Winitz, 1975). However, discrimination training may not directly improve production ability. Williams and McReynolds (1975) studied discrimination and production training in an alternating treatments design. Their results indicated that discrimination training resulted in improved discrimination scores but did not influence the production scores. In contrast, production training resulted in improved scores in both production and discrimination. These results raise a question about the necessity of discrimination training. In fact, it is not clear that all children have difficulty with discrimination, even of their own error sounds (Locke, 1980a). More research is needed to clarify the role of auditory discrimination training in phonological remediation. As seen in Chapter 3, little is known about the role of perception relative to production in normal children; this is also true for disordered children. Until more definitive information is available, auditory training tasks might be viewed as a "training variable" to use in conjunction with production work (Shelton and McReynolds, 1979).

There are a variety of techniques that offer alternatives to auditory discrimination tasks. For example, Weiner and Bankson (1978) described an auditory "sorting" task in which contrasting words were grouped into categories based on the phonetic characteristics of the phonemes in the words (e.g., continuant versus noncontinuant). Hodson and Paden's (1983) technique of auditory bombardment is another example of presenting the child with controlled listening experiences. Yet another technique is auditory self-monitoring, a task in which a child produces the target unit and then judges its accuracy.

The ability to judge one's productions at a conscious level is possibly essential for improvement and long-term maintenance of sound production (Shelton and McReynolds, 1979; Shriberg and Kwiatkowski, 1982a). However, self-monitoring is not an easy skill to develop; it is a sophisticated metalinguistic task that requires good memory and some ability to segment words into sounds. A study by Ruscello and Shelton (1979) that incorporated self-monitoring shows the difficulty of this task. Their teaching paradigm combined the techniques of planning how to produce the target sound and then judging the accuracy of the production. They found that whereas the 7-year-olds in the treatment group made more improvement than the control group they were essentially unsuccessful at recognizing their incorrect responses. However, these authors did not report whether they taught the children how to judge their own errors. Perhaps children must not only be cognitively mature enough to carry out the task (possibly 6–7 years old), but must also be taught how to respond to such a task.

In summary, this brief discussion of auditory training emphasizes a few salient issues. There are several types of auditory training, and the relationship between the various types of training and production ability is not clear. Not all children necessarily benefit from auditory training, so it is important to select the auditory training task based on a child's specific abilities. Techniques such as auditory bombardment and self-monitoring must be studied empirically in order to understand their role in phonological remediation.

Contextual Facilitation The use of the phonetic context as a means of facilitating production is another technique that can be incorporated into remediation. There has been empirical study of the effects of phonetic context on accuracy of production (Gallagher and Shriner, 1975; Hoffman et al., 1980), but these results have not been integrated with treatment that is linguistically based. This lack of integration reflects the dichotomy of viewing speech errors as either motoric or linguistic. Use of facilitating contexts in conjunction with conceptual activities could very well result in more rapid progress in therapy.

Kent (1982) illustrated the value of incorporating contextual information into treatment. He identified four major factors that could facilitate production. First, he suggested working on sounds in *stressed syllables* because they require more precise articulatory placement, which in turn gives the child clearer auditory feedback. In addition, practicing a sound in a particular *word or syllable position* may facilitate production, e.g., /s/ in word-final position; the most appropriate position varies according to the child and the sound. *Sounds adjacent to the target sound* can be facilitative if they either present minimal interference with the target sound or are very similar to the features of the target, e.g., [t] facilitates [s] in the context [st]. Finally, the *type of error* a child demonstrates (e.g., dentalization or lateralization of [s]) affects what sort of facilitating context is chosen. Kent suggested that each child be tested to determine which of the above factors can be used to enhance performance. Articulatory and acoustic features serve as the best guidelines for selection of cues to test.

Definition of a Correct Response and Criteria for Sound Mastery

An important feature of some phonological treatment programs is the definition of a correct response. Instead of accepting only the target sound as correct, some authors (Ingram, 1976; Weiner, 1981b) suggested accepting any production that falls within the sound class. This procedure was used in a phonological process study completed by Weiner (1981b). He accepted any fricative production as appropriate because it eliminated the substitution of stops for fricatives. The justification to accept approximations is based on two sources. First, studies of normal acquisition indicate that children usually progress gradually through stages as they acquire correct sound production. Second, clinicians often accept approximations of the correct response as one step toward mastery of a sound. Accepting productions that are not correct but that are in the desired sound class assumes that the child will eventually recognize the error and spontaneously produce the correct sound. Some children may be able to do this without further training, and others may not. The definition of a correct response must be investigated with many children in order to understand how the concept can be used most effectively in phonological remediation.

Related to the issue of whether a sound must be trained until it is produced correctly is the issue of whether a sound must be trained to mastery. Traditionally, a sound is trained until it is correctly produced in approximately 90% of the possible occurrences in continuous speech. However, it may not be necessary to train a sound to this level. For example, Hodson and Paden (1983) suggested that lengthy practice is not essential. Auditory stimulation and intensive production practice for a short time may be sufficient to stimulate emergence and eventual mastery. In order to determine how much training is necessary, children must be taught to a particular level of production accuracy and then monitored to determine if they can maintain and master the correct production without further training.

In a study concerning criteria for sound mastery, Olswang and Bain (1982) investigated the following question: "How much treatment is necessary and sufficient for stimulating the acquisition of a phoneme so that therapy on that sound can be terminated as early as possible?" These children were taught the production of target consonants through a traditional hierarchy (isolation, syllables, words, phrases, and sentences). Treatment was terminated when the children produced the target phoneme at one of the following three criterion levels in untrained words:

1. Three consecutive data points reflecting a stable upward or flat trend of 30–74% correct production
2. Two consecutive data points reflecting a stable upward or flat trend of 75–99% correct production
3. A single data point of 100% correct production

After treatment was terminated on a phoneme, productions were monitored to determine if high levels of accuracy (75–100% correct) were maintained.

As seen in Table 7.3, training for the eight sounds was terminated at criterion levels 1, 2, or 3, described above. The percentage of correct production in untrained words at the termination of therapy is also presented in Table 7.3. For the first six of the sounds, production levels remained high and additional treatment was not necessary. Production levels of the last two sounds (initial /s/ and final /l/ for S3) dropped after training was terminated. Treatment was reinstated briefly for these two sounds; performance improved and continued to be high. The authors concluded that for some sounds and some children treatment can be

Table 7.3 Criteria and Percentages for Termination of Treatment

Criteria for Termination	Sounds Achieving Criterion Level	Percentage of Correct Production at Termination
30–74%	f- (S1)[a]	40
	g- (S2)	40
	l- (S3)	63
75–100%	l- (S1)	100
	-l (S1)	78
	l- (S2)	100
	s- (S3)	88, 75[b]
	-l (S3)	88, 88[b]

From Olswang and Bain (1982).
[a]Chronological age for the subjects was: S1, 4;0; S2, 4;5; and S3, 4;9.
[b]Treatment was reintroduced for these two sounds.

terminated rather rapidly, whereas for other sounds and children more prolonged treatment is required. It is important to be able to predict both situations. Olswang and Bain (1982) made the following observations regarding factors that might lead to predictions:

1. The child who required more treatment (S3) demonstrated some oral motor involvement.
2. This child had more inconsistent substitutions than the other children.
3. Successful termination of treatment was usually preceded by correct production of the sound in a variety of phonetic contexts in continuous speech.

This study is valuable because it identified variables that may have a role in successful sound acquisition. Each of these observations should be studied systematically, so that criteria for terminating treatment on a sound can be developed. The results of this study suggest that training to a high level of accurate production in continuous speech may not be necessary for many children or for all sounds.

Measurement of Treatment Effectiveness

Many factors have been identified in this chapter that are thought to influence normal acquisition of the phonological system, and many approaches and techniques have been proposed to facilitate acquisition in disordered children. Unfortunately, we still have numerous unanswered questions about how to develop the most appropriate treatment procedures for different errors and children. In the face of many questions and few answers, each speech-language clinician must choose among approaches and techniques to accomplish the most effective and efficient treatment possible. These choices should be based on as much quantified information as possible. That is, the clinician must measure or test treatment effectiveness.

The purpose of this measurement is to: (1) identify variables that succeed or fail in making changes in phonological behavior; and (2) measure the generalization of trained responses to untrained linguistic content and situations. There are certain principles of measurement that can guide this procedure. One consideration is *what* to measure. It is important to measure the child's accuracy with *trained* as well as *untrained* stimuli. Trained stimuli should be tested within the treatment setting and at school or at home. This measurement can reflect the success or failure of the treatment techniques; if there is a lack of progress, changes can systematically be made until success is achieved. The second aspect of measurement involves testing untrained stimuli—including (1) other sounds within the sound class; (2) new lexical items; (3) different word positions; and (4) continuous speech—in order to determine if the child is generalizing the trained response. Again, if generalization is not occurring, modifications can be made in the treatment approach to help the child become aware of additional ways to use the new abilities. For example, a child may be successful in producing words with initial /k/ in a variety of activities and settings (i.e., success with trained stimuli), but does not produce /k/ in untrained words or continuous speech and does not produce other velar sounds (i.e., lack of successful response generalization). From these results the clinician can assume that treatment techniques were successful in establishing the target behavior but that the child needs help with generalization.

Procedures for measuring treatment effectiveness involve setting aside a short period of time for presentation of the trained or untrained stimuli. The child typically receives no teaching cues or reinforcement; in other words, the measurement is like a test. The most typical stimuli for measuring progress are trained and untrained words and continuous speech. Therefore the child is given an opportunity to produce the words without feedback and to interact and converse for a short period (e.g., 3–5 min). Measurement should be done at consistent, frequent intervals (every 7–10 days), in order to use the information to make decisions about ongoing treatment effectiveness. The measurement procedures do take time to administer, but they are essential if we are to understand more clearly the reasons why our treatment procedures do and do not work.

Summary

The treatment variables discussed in this section included reference to linguistic, cognitive, auditory, and motoric factors. The range of these variables makes it clear that phonological remediation must incorporate information from a variety of domains. It is limiting to address one aspect of the system, e.g., linguistic skills, while ignoring another, e.g., motoric learning. Clinical treatment programs and empirical studies must incorporate all of the domains in order to provide the most effective treatment program. A framework that integrates the selection of linguistic content to be taught with the structure of the session and techniques for presenting the content will be most likely to meet the needs of individual children.

Conclusions

Phonological remediation currently incorporates such concepts as distinctive features, phonological processes, contrast, and generalization. Remediation programs are sometimes described as "conceptual" because the goal is to teach the child to use sounds in a meaningful, contrastive way. Consequently, treatment sessions tend to be less structured, because there is more opportunity for interaction between the child and clinician. There is currently less active interest in traditional ideas, e.g., auditory and motoric training and operant conditioning techniques. In many ways there is a lack of integration between the newer phonological concepts and the more traditional concepts. This lack of integration seems to be the result of three factors.

The first factor relates to the tendency for researchers and clinicians to adopt a currently popular view or position and apply it almost exclusively to treatment. This has been apparent with the application of operant conditioning techniques during the 1960s, distinctive feature training programs during the early 1970s, and most recently the application of phonological processes to assessment and treatment. It is critical that new concepts be systematically incorporated into treatment, but it is equally important to integrate newer concepts with existing, well-documented concepts.

Another factor that makes integration of concepts difficult is the knowledge base that exists for normal and disordered child phonology. Much information is lacking about acquisition, particularly in the areas of perception and motor skills. There is much to learn about how and when phonological processes are used by normal children and about the mastery of the phonological system from 2 to 4 years of age. Information about acquisition is available from a variety of sources; but it is only gradually that this information filters into speech pathology, first into assessment procedures and later into treatment procedures. Given that clinicians must integrate extremely complex information from a variety of sources and apply it to treatment, it is not surprising that there is a lack of integration across the domains that relate to disordered phonology.

Finally, there is a lack of integration in phonological remediation because of the lack of a model for treatment. There is no agreement about the essential behaviors that should be evaluated and taught or the approaches that would best achieve those behaviors. Although there is no empirical data base to support it, it is beneficial to formulate a hypothetical model that can be used as a basis for planning and implementing treatment. As new data are obtained, the model and the treatment plan can be refined. Such a model could serve an integrative function, to allow the clinician and researcher to consider cognitive, linguistic, perceptual, and motoric factors simultaneously as they relate to disordered phonology.

Chapter 8

Conclusion

In the first chapter we identified a number of issues we believe are particularly important for understanding normal and disordered phonological development. We return to those issues in this chapter in order to sum up our current knowledge of each. In addition, we include some suggestions regarding directions for future research in the area of phonological development and disorders.

Current Issues Revisited

Universal Patterns Versus Individual Differences

The crux of the issue of universal patterns versus individual differences as stated in Chapter 1, was whether phonological development proceeds along a universal and presumably innate course, or whether each child follows his or her own idiosyncratic path. Given the data presented in Chapters 2 and 3, it should now be obvious that this issue cannot be considered as an *either/or* question. Phonological development is based on both universal or near-universal patterns and idiosyncratic strategies formulated by each child. The universal patterns can be attributed to the nature of the human auditory and articulatory systems and to the effects of

195

maturation. The idiosyncratic aspects of acquisition are best accounted for by cognitive factors involving the recognition, storage, retrieval, and production of words in the ambient language.

The existence of individual differences in phonological development makes it all the more difficult to identify children with a phonological disorder. If we accept the idea that children can differ substantially in their patterns of acquisition, how do we decide that a given child is displaying an atypical pattern? This is an area for future research: investigations aimed at defining the *range* of individual differences in normally developing children are essential as a basis for identifying children who fall outside that range.

Another aspect of individual differences that needs to be studied relates to age. Research to date suggests that the differences are greatest in the initial stages of acquisition, and that for the most part they are greatly diminished (or have disappeared) by the age of 3;6–4;0. If this observation holds true, it will greatly facilitate the task of distinguishing children with acquisition patterns within the normal range from those exhibiting disordered patterns.

Factors Underlying Mispronunciations

In Chapter 1 it was noted that failure to pronounce a word correctly could be attributed to a number of factors including: (1) lack of motor ability to *articulate* a particular sound or sound sequence; (2) failure to *perceive* the word accurately; (3) failure to *remember* (i.e., store) the pronunciation accurately: (4) a *production constraint* on the general form of all words (e.g., no word can end in a consonant); (5) a *lack of knowledge* about the phonological system of the adult language (e.g., a child might not "know" that /s/ and /ʃ/ are distinct phonemes in English, and consequently might treat them as variants of a single phoneme); and (6) any combination of the above. Identification of the cause(s) of pronunciation errors is particularly important for children with a phonological disorder, because effective treatment plans for these children should depend, in large part, on the nature of the underlying cause.

Phonological process analyses such as those presented in Chapter 4 are valuable for comparing adult and child pronunciations and for identifying error patterns on the part of the child. However, they are only a first step in determining underlying causes—they provide a *description* but not an *explanation* of pronunciation errors. Consider, for example, the normally developing child SR (described in Chapter 4), who regularly omitted unstressed syllables in word-initial position. We can describe her error pattern as the process of Unstressed Syllable Deletion, but naming the error pattern is not enough. We must also try to explain it: Does SR omit unstressed syllables because they are difficult to perceive, difficult to produce, or both? Perhaps she perceives unstressed syllables but fails to include them in her underlying representations, i.e., her *stored* form of the words.

Explanations of pronunciation errors cannot be based solely on analysis of a transcribed speech sample or the results of an articulation test; transcription-based analyses must be supplemented by assessments of articulatory skills, auditory discrimination and linguistic perception, and a child's underlying representations. In addition, longitudinal data are necessary to identify frozen forms and to determine the rate and direction of change; and acoustic analyses are needed to identify phonemic distinctions that may be present but are imperceptible to adult listeners.

In reality, it is not always possible to obtain all the types of information desired. Assessing linguistic perception, for example, is not easy, and the findings may not be clear-cut (see Chapter 3 for a discussion); even more difficult is figuring out a child's underlying representation for a mispronounced word or set of words. Several techniques have been suggested (e.g., Dinnsen et al., 1979; Locke, 1980b; Macken, 1980b), all of which are time-consuming and none of which are entirely satisfactory. In spite of the difficulties involved in gathering and assessing data related to the causes of pronunciation errors, both researchers and clinicians must be aware that in order to *explain* (rather than describe) they must consider an array of factors in addition to a transcribed speech sample. To date, studies of disordered children have given more attention to these factors than studies of normal children, which tend to be primarily descriptive. In the future, the emphasis of research should be on explanation, as well as description, for both populations.

Units of Acquisition

It was suggested in Chapter 1 that phonological development may not involve simply the learning of phonemes and distinctive features but, in the early stages, the learning of whole words and/or syllables. In other words, learning may involve different *units* of acquisition at different developmental stages. Evidence in support of the notion that at least some words are acquired as indivisible wholes comes from a variety of sources.

First, it was noted (Chapter 2) that in the "first 50 word" stage, production patterns seemed to involve *words* rather than segments, as shown by a lack of systematic error patterns based on single sounds or sound classes. Second, the occurrence of words that do not conform to the rest of the child's phonological system, either because they are pronounced more accurately (*advanced forms*) or less accurately (*frozen forms*) than expected, indicates that they are unanalyzed units. When such words change so that they conform to the system, we can hypothesize that they have been broken down into their component parts. Finally, examples such as those presented by Waterson (1971), in which a set of words with shared phonetic and structural features is produced with a single output pattern (e.g., *finger, Randall, another, window* were all pronounced alike), provide more evidence of a "whole-word" approach. The child does not attempt to produce the exact segments of the adult words but, rather, to reproduce the "salient" features of the target words—in this case, the features nasal and disyllabic.

Although there seems to be sufficient evidence to conclude that there is more than one unit of acquisition, our understanding of the various units is far from complete. Questions that should be pursued include: Do all children go through a "whole-word" stage before a phonemic stage? When does the transition from one stage to another occur? Do all words undergo a reanalysis at the same time? If not, why? Do children with phonological disorders behave differently in this domain? Research directed toward these questions will increase our understanding of phonological development in general.

Nature of Disordered Phonology

In Chapter 1 the discussion of disordered phonology raised the possibility of identifying subgroups of children with phonological disorders. It was suggested, for example, that children be classified as either *delayed* or *deviant* on the basis of their pronunciation patterns. If their productions resembled those of younger, normally developing children, they would be considered "delayed." If their speech patterns were qualitatively different from those of normal children, however, they would be classified as "deviant."

Although these categories seem to be a logical means of forming subgroups, they have not proved adequate. As discussed in Chapter 5, children with a disordered phonological system cannot be easily placed into a category of deviancy or delay, because most of them display speech patterns associated with both categories. For example, their inventories of segmental phones and syllabic structures are likely to include a high proportion of stops, nasals, and glides, as well as simple syllabic types, e.g., CV or CVC. In this regard, their productions resemble those of young, normal children. At the same time, however, the disordered children may incorporate *idiosyncratic* processes into their speech (i.e., processes that rarely occur in the productions of normal children), making their productions very different from those of children with normally developing phonological systems. In addition, disordered children may evidence a Chronological Mismatch in terms of the order of acquisition of phonemes; that is, they may correctly pronounce some phonemes that are typically acquired late while failing to produce other phonemes usually acquired early. The idiosyncratic features of the speech of disordered children tend to make pronunciation patterns differ substantially across the population. As shown in Chapter 6, two children, both of whom are classified as having "severe" phonological disorders, can have very distinct phonological systems. In the case at hand, the speech of neither child met the description of being "delayed" or "deviant." Thus although there may be subgroups of disordered children, the delayed/deviant dichotomy does not adequately characterize disordered phonology. Further research is required to determine if disordered children can be grouped according to their patterns of speech production or by some other aspect of their speech.

In Chapter 5 it was suggested that phonological disorders could be characterized as a disorder involving the *process* of acquisition, thereby creating atypical patterns associated with the *product* of acquisition. According to this view, children with a phonological disorder proceed through the course of acquisition differently from normal children. In particular, children with phonological disorders seem to adhere to a different timetable for the emergence and mastery of sounds and for the occurrence and suppression of phonological processes. For example, a disordered child may use a phonological process, e.g., Final Consonant Deletion (which typically disappears fairly early), at the same time that his phonetic inventory expands rapidly. As a result, the child would have a wide range of phones but a severely restricted range of syllabic types, creating a system quite different from that of a normal child.

The view that phonological disorders involve the *process* of acquisition (i.e., the *way* children approach and/or proceed through the acquisition process) is largely untested. Future research on a range of disordered populations will provide data to support or refute this idea. If the view is supported, the next step is to attempt to relate etiological factors to abnormal patterns in the process of acquisition.

Generalization

Generalization was introduced as an important issue because it is usually cited as one of the fundamental goals of remediation. Although it is clearly a desirable goal, so far remediation techniques aimed at enhancing generalization have not been very promising (see Chapter 7). The failure may be due, at least in part, to the (unwarranted) assumption that a trained response automatically generalizes to new linguistic contexts and new settings. Because this assumption cannot be made, it is the responsibility of the clinician to facilitate generalization by developing a teaching approach that: (1) encourages self-monitoring; (2) gives the client the responsibility for change; and (3) includes other people and settings from the beginning of treatment.

If generalization does not occur with this approach, the approach must be modified so that the client begins to generalize. Generalization does not occur automatically—it is *not* a passive phenomenon. Rather, it must be considered a basic element of the remediation plan. As clinicians (and researchers) systematically monitor whether generalization is occurring, they can begin to predict when it will (and will not) take place. For example, after observing a group of children with a particular error pattern (e.g., velar fronting), we will have some idea if training on a single sound (e.g., on /k/) is sufficient for generalization or if each sound in the velar class will have to be trained. On the basis of systematic studies of success and failure, we should be able to derive some general principles regarding ways of enhancing generalization in disordered children.

At the same time that we strive for a better understanding of this phenomenon, we must bear in mind that the most consistent result of empirical studies carried out to date is that children differ greatly in their ability to generalize. Future research, then, should be directed not only toward the development of techniques that will increase the likelihood of generalization but also toward an understanding of the differences in children's abilities to generalize.

Future Research

Although our understanding of normal and disordered phonological development has increased substantially during the past decade, it is far from complete and many unanswered questions remain. Some of these have already been mentioned in this chapter; in fact, our discussion of each of the issues (individual differences, factors underlying mispronunciations, units of acquisition, the nature of phonological disorders, and generalization) includes suggestions for research aimed at furthering our understanding of the particular issue. In addition, there are two areas that, although not cited as "current issues," we believe should be targeted for future investigations.

Input

We know very little about the phonological characteristics of speech addressed to children and even less about the effects of that speech on phonological acquisition (see Chapter 3). Both aspects of input deserve more attention in the future. In particular we should attempt to identify which features of input (if any) may facilitate acquisition. Features to be considered include slow speech, careful articulation, repetition, limited vocabulary of phonologically simple words, etc. At the same time, there may be factors that hinder acquisition by confusing the child, e.g., variable pronunciation of a target word, rapid speech, dialectic differences, etc. At present, the occurrence and importance of these factors have not been systematically investigated. It is our hope that future research will provide answers to questions in this area.

Early Identification of a Disorder

At what age can phonological disorders be identified? In most cases, they are not identified until a child is 3–4 years old, sometimes even older. By this age, pronunciation patterns may be relatively fixed and consequently are more difficult to remediate.

Research aimed at the early identification of phonological disorders would be a valuable contribution, particularly in the clinical area. We should start by going back to the earliest vocalizations—those of the babbling stage—and attempt to determine if some babies exhibit atypical production patterns during this period. If so, these babies would be designated as "at risk" for the subsequent development of a disorder. If no differences are found at the babbling stage (and research to date suggests that this is the case), then we should consider the initial stage of the linguistic period—the first 50 words.

Investigation of this stage should focus on aspects that might be associated with a phonological disorder. These might include: (1) age at onset of meaningful speech; (2) rate of acquisition of the first words; (3) pronunciation patterns evident in the first words; and (4) oral motoric abilities. Given the wide range of behaviors reported for children designated as "normal" during the "first 50 word" stage, it is difficult to imagine what would constitute an atypical pattern, but one (or more) might be identified from studies involving large numbers of subjects.

An important factor relating to early identification of a disorder involves the medical history of children who might be considered "at risk." For example, it has been shown that children with recurrent otitis media (inflammation of the middle ear) before the age of 2 have a higher incidence of phonological disorders than those who have not had otitis media. Otitis-prone children, then, are obvious candidates for early intervention if their speech patterns seem to be developing slowly or in an atypical fashion.

In sum, early identification of phonological disorders is an area that clearly needs further attention. Such research will contribute to our understanding of normal as well as disordered development.

Conclusion

Our current understanding of the major issues highlighted in Chapter 1 is summed up in this chapter. As we said initially, it was not our intention to provide hard-and-fast answers to any of the questions. However, we did attempt to construct a framework that allows the issues to be considered from various points of view. In so doing, we have raised many new questions that merit further attention. In addition, we have identified two other topics that we feel are crucial areas for future research.

We join others in the field (e.g., Locke, 1983a; Smith, 1981) in stressing the need for investigations directed toward *explaining* rather than *describing* phonological development and disorders. Descriptions are, of course, an important part of research in these areas, but they are only a first step. They must be complemented by studies and theories aimed at explaining the phenomena that have been described.

Appendix A

Segmental Symbols

Table A.1 Consonants

	Bilabial	Labiodental	Dental	Alveolar	Lateral	Alveolo-palatal	Palatal	Velar	Uvular	Pharyngeal	Glottal
Stop											
– Voice	p	p̪	t̪	t	—	—	c	k	q	—	ʔ
+ Voice	b	b̪	d̪	d	—	—	ɟ	g	ɢ	—	—
Fricative											
– Voice	ɸ	f	θ	s	ɬ	ʃ	ç	x	χ	ħ	h
+ Voice	β	v	ð	z	ɮ	ʒ	ʝ	ɣ	ʁ	ʕ	ɦ
Affricate											
– Voice	p͡ɸ	p͡f	t͡θ	t͡s	t͡ɬ	t͡ʃ	c͡ç	k͡x	q͡χ	q͡ħ	ʔ͡h
+ Voice	b͡β	b͡v	d͡ð	d͡z	d͡ɮ	d͡ʒ	ɟ͡ʝ	g͡ɣ	ɢ͡ʁ	g͡ʕ	ʔ͡ɦ
Nasal (+ voice)	m	ɱ	n̪	n	—	—	ɲ	ŋ	ɴ	—	—
Liquid (+ voice)	—			r	l	—	ʎ	ɫ			
Trill (+ voice)	B			r̃					R		
Flap (+ voice)	—			ɾ					ɽ		
Glides (+ voice)	w ʍ ʍ						j				unpursed r-like

205

Table A.2 Vowels

	Front		Central		Back	
	− rnd	+ rnd	− rnd	+ rnd	− rnd	+ rnd
High {	i ɪ	y	ɨ	ʉ	ɯ	u ʊ
Mid {	e ɛ	ø œ	ə ʌ	ɚ ɝ	ɤ	o ɔ
Low	æ		a		ɑ	

Appendix B

Diacritics

Description	Symbol	Example(s)
Labialized	[͜]	[s̫]
Dentalized	[̩]	[s̩]
Bladed	[̺]	[ḏ] [s̺]
Palatalized	[ʸ]	[tʸ] [sʸ]
Retroflexed	[..]	[t̤]
Voiced	[ᵥ]	[f̬]
Devoiced	[̥]	[m̥] [o̥]
Nasalized	[˜]	[õ]
Denasalized	[˟]	[ń]
Aspirated (stop)	[ʰ]	[tʰ]
Unreleased (stop)	[˥]	[t˥]
Tongue body advanced	[←]	[a←]
Tongue body retracted	[→]	[a→]
Tongue body raised	[↑]	[a↑]
Tongue body lowered	[↓]	[a↓]
Weakened articulation	Small raised segment	[ᵖfu] [oʳ]
Lengthened segment	[:]	[m:] [a:]
Syllabic consonant	[ˌ]	[n̩] [l̩]
Syllable boundary	[,]	[o,a]
Primary stress	[ʹ]	[əʹbaʊt]

207

References

Allen, G. D. 1976. Development of rhythm in early phonology. Paper presented at Eighth Annual Child Language Research Forum, April, Stanford, CA.

Allen, G. D. 1977. On transcribing the American r. Paper presented at the Joint IPS-77/AAPS Meeting, Miami Beach.

Allen, G. D., and **Hawkins, S.** 1980. Phonological rhythm: definition and development. In: G. Yeni-Komshian, J. F. Kavanagh, and C. A. Ferguson (eds.), Child Phonology, Vol. 1, pp. 227–256. Academic Press, New York.

Aram, D., and **Kamhi, A.** 1982. Perspectives on the relationship between phonological and language disorders. Semin. Speech Lang. Hear. 3:101–114.

Arthur, G. 1952. The Arthur Adaptation of the Leiter International Performance Scale. Psychological Service Center Press, Washington, DC.

Atkinson, K., MacWhinney, B., and **Stoel, C.** 1968. An experiment on the recognition of babbling. Working Paper 15, Language Behavior Research Laboratory, University of California, Berkeley.

Bank, R., Hanrahan, L., and **Langlois, A.** 1983. The relationship between children's use of phonological processes and the syntactical complexity of their utterances. Paper presented at the 18th Mid-America Linguistics Conference. October 14–15, Boulder, CO.

Barton, D. 1975. Statistical significance in phonemic perception experiments. J. Child Lang. 2:297–298.

Barton, D. 1976. The role of perception in the acquisition of phonology. Doctoral dissertation, London. Indiana University Linguistics Club, Bloomington.

Barton, D. 1980. Phonemic perception in children. In: G. Yeni-Komshian, J. F. Kavanagh, and C. A. Ferguson (eds.), Child Phonology, Vol. 2, pp. 97–116. Academic Press, New York.

Benedict, H. 1979. Early lexical development: comprehension and production. J. Child Lang. 6:183–200.

Bernstein-Ratner, N. 1983. Increased vowel precision in the absence of increased vowel duration. Paper presented at the annual meeting of the American Speech-Language-Hearing Association, November 18–21, Cincinnati.

Bernthal, J., and **Bankson, N.** 1981. Articulation Disorders. Prentice-Hall, New York.

Blache, S., Parsons, C., and **Humphreys, J.** 1981. A minimal-word-pair model for teaching the linguistic significance of distinctive feature properties. J. Speech Hear. Res. 46:291–296.

Bloom, L. 1973. One Word at a Time. Mouton, The Hague.

Bloom, L. M., Hood, L., and **Lightbown, P.** 1974., Imitation in language development: if, when and why. Cognitive Psychol. 6:380–420.

Braine, M. D. S. 1974. On what might constitute learnable phonology. Language 50:270–299.

Braine, M. D. S. 1976. Review of N. V. Smith, The Acquisition of Phonology. Language 52:489–498.

Branigan, G. 1977. Some early constraints on word combinations. Unpublished doctoral dissertation, Boston University.

Bright, W. 1976. Variation and Change in Language: Essays by William Bright. Stanford University Press, Stanford, CA.

Brown, R. 1958. Words and Things. Free Press, Glencoe, IL.

Brown, R. 1973. A First Language. Harvard University Press, Cambridge, MA.

Brown, R., and **Bellugi, U.** 1964. Three processes in the child's acquisition of syntax. Harvard Educ. Rev. 34:133–151.

Carrow, E. 1973. Test for Auditory Comprehension of Language. Urban Research Group, Austin, TX.

Carrow, E. 1974. Carrow Elicited Language Inventory. Learning Concepts, Austin, TX.

Carter, A. 1974. The development of communication in the sensorimotor period: a case study. Unpublished doctoral dissertation, University of California, Berkeley.

Carter, A. 1979. Prespeech meaning relations: an outline of one infant's sensorimotor morpheme development. In: P. Fletcher and M. Garman (eds.), Language Acquisition, pp. 71–92. Cambridge University Press, Cambridge.

Carter, E., and **Buck, M.** 1958. Prognostic testing for functional articulation disorders among children in the first grade. J. Speech Hear. Disord. 23:124–133.

Chomsky, N., and **Halle, M.** 1968. The Sound Pattern of English. Harper & Row, New York.

Clumeck, H. 1977. Topics in the acquisition of Mandarin phonology: a case study. Papers Rep. Child Lang. Dev. 14:37–73.

Clumeck, H. 1982. The effect of word familiarity on phonemic recognition in preschool children aged 3 to 5 years. In: C. E. Johnson and C. L. Thew (eds.), Proceedings of the Second International Congress for the Study of Child Language, Vol. 1, pp. 58–77. University Press of America, Washington, DC.

Compton, A. J. 1970. Generative studies of children's phonological disorders. J. Speech Hear. Disord. 35:315–339.

Compton, A. 1976. Generative studies of children's phonological disorders: clinical ramifications. In: D. Morehead and A. Morehead (eds.), Normal and Deficient Child Language, pp. 61–96. University Park Press, Baltimore.

Costello, J. 1977. Programmed instruction. J. Speech Hear. Disord. 42:3–28.

Costello, J., and Onstine, J. 1976. The modification of multiple articulation errors based on distinctive feature theory. J. Speech Hear. Disord. 41:199–215.

Crary, M., Wellmers, T., and Blache, S. 1981. A preliminary look at phonological process suppression. Paper presented at the Second International Congress for the Study of Child Language, August 9–14. Vancouver, BC.

Crocker, J. 1969. A phonological model of children's articulation competence. J. Speech Hear. Disord. 34:203–213.

Dinnsen, D. A. 1984. Methods and empirical issues in analyzing functional misarticulation. In: M. Elbert, D. A. Dinnsen, and G. Weismer (eds.), Phonological Theory and the Misarticulating Child. ASHA Monogr. 22:5–17.

Dinnsen, D. A., Elbert, M., and Weismer, G. 1979. On the characterization of functional misarticulations. Paper presented at the annual convention of the American Speech-Language-Hearing Association, November 21–23, Atlanta.

Donegan, P. J., and Stampe, D. 1979. The study of natural phonology. In: D. A. Dinnsen (ed.), Current Approaches to Phonological Theory, pp. 126–173. Indiana University Press, Bloomington.

Dore, J., Franklin, M. B., Miller, R. T., and Ramer, A. L. 1976. Transitional phenomena in early language acquisition. J. Child Lang. 3:13–28.

Dubois, E. M., and Bernthal, J. E. 1978. A comparison of three methods for obtaining articulatory responses. J. Speech Hear. Disord. 43:295–305.

Dunn, C. 1982. Phonological process analysis: contributions to assessing phonological disorders. Commun. Disord. 7:147–163.

Dunn, C. 1983. Production of multisyllabic words by phonologically disordered children. Proceedings from the Fourth Wisconsin Symposium on Research in Child Language Disorders. University of Wisconsin, Madison.

Dunn, C., and Barron, C. 1982. A treatment program for disordered phonology: phonetic and linguistic considerations. Lang. Speech Hear. Serv. Schools 13:100–109.

Dunn, C., and Davis, B. 1983. Phonological process occurrence in phonologically disordered children. Appl. Psycholing. 4:187–207.

Dunn, C., Richardson, A., Davis, B., and Newton, L. 1983. An interaction model for treatment of language and phonological disorders. Paper presented at the annual convention of the Speech-Language-Hearing Association, November 18–21, Cincinnati.

Dunn, C., and Till, J. 1982. Morphophonemic rule learning in normal and articulation-disordered children. J. Speech Hear. Res. 25:322–333.

Dunn, L. 1981. Peabody Picture Vocabulary Test—Revised. American Guidance Service, Circle Pines, MN.

Eady, S. 1980. The onset of language-specific patterning in infant vocalization. MA thesis, University of Ottawa.

Edwards, M. L. 1974. Perception and production in child phonology: the testing of four hypotheses. J. Child Lang. 1:205–219.

Edwards, M. L. 1978. Word position in fricative acquisition. Paper presented at the Boston University Conference on Language Acquisition, Boston.

Edwards, M. L. 1979. Patterns and processes in fricative acquisition: longitudinal evidence from six English-learning children. Unpublished doctoral dissertation, Stanford University.

Edwards, M. L. 1980a. Phonological analysis of children's speech. Paper presented at the Annual Convention of the American Speech-Language-Hearing Association, Detroit.

Edwards, M. L. 1980b. The use of "favorite sounds" by children with phonological disorders. Paper presented at the Fifth Annual Boston University Conference on Language Development, October, Boston.

Edwards, M., and Bernhardt, B. 1973. Phonological analyses of the speech of four children with language disorders. Unpublished manuscript from the Institute for Childhood Aphasia, Stanford University.

Eguchi, S., and Hirsch, I. J. 1969. Development of speech sounds in children. Acta Otolaryngol. [Suppl] (Stockh) 257.

Eilers, R. E., and Minifie, F. 1975. Fricative discrimination in early infancy. J. Speech Hear. Res. 18:158–167.

Eilers, R. E., and Oller, D. K. 1976. The role of speech discrimination in developmental sound substitutions. J. Child Lang. 3:319–329.

Eilers, R., Wilson, W., and Moore, J. 1977. Developmental changes in speech discrimination in infants. J. Speech Hear. Res. 20:766–780.

Eimas, P. D. 1974. Auditory and linguistic processing of cues for places of articulation by infants. Perception Psychophys. 16:513–521.

Eimas, P., Siqueland, E. R., Jusczyk, P., and Vigorito, J. 1971. Speech perception in infants. Science 171:303–306.

Elbert, M., and McReynolds, L. 1978. An experimental analysis of misarticulating children's generalization. J. Speech Hear. Disord. 21:136–150.

Elbert, M., Rockmann, B., and Saltzman, D. 1980. Contrasts: The Use of Minimal Pairs in Articulation Training. Exceptional Resources, Austin, TX.

Faircloth, M., and Faircloth, S. 1970. An analysis of the articulatory behavior of a speech-defective child in connected speech and in isolated-word responses. J. Speech Hear. Disord. 35:51–61.

Farquhar, M. 1961. Prognostic value of imitative and auditory discrimination tests. J. Speech Hear. Disord. 26:342–347.

Farwell, C. B. 1977. Some strategies in the early production of fricatives. Papers Rep. Child Lang. 12:97–104.

Fee, J., and Ingram, D. 1982. Reduplication as a strategy of phonological development. J. Child Lang. 9:41–54.

Ferguson, C. A. 1964. Baby talk in six languages. Am. Anthropol. 64:103–114.

Ferguson, C. A. 1968. Contrastive analysis and language development. Georgetown Univ. Monogr. Ser. Lang. Linguistics 21:101–112.

Ferguson, C. A. 1975. Fricatives in child language acquisition. In: Proceedings of the Eleventh International Congress of Linguists, Bologna–Florence, pp. 647–664.

Ferguson, C. A. 1978. Learning to pronounce: the earliest stages of phonological development in the child. In: F. D. Minifie and L. L. Lloyd (eds.), Communicative Competence and Cognitive Abilities, pp. 237–297. University Park Press, Baltimore.

Ferguson, C. A. 1983. Reduplication in child phonology. J. Child Lang. 10:239–244.

Ferguson, C. A., and Farwell, C. B. 1975. Words and sounds in early language acquisition: English initial consonants in the first fifty words. Language 51:419–439.

Ferguson, C. A., and Garnica, O. K. 1975. Theories of phonological development. In: E. Lenneberg and E. Lenneberg (eds.), Foundations of Language Development, pp. 153–180. Academic Press, New York.

Ferguson, C. A., Peizer, D. B., and Weeks, T. E. 1973. Model-and-replica phonological grammar of a child's first words. Lingua 31:35–65.

Ferguson, C. A., and Yeni-Komshian, G. 1980. An introduction to speech production in the child. In: G. Yeni-Komshian, J. A. Kavanagh, and C. A. Ferguson (eds.), Child Phonology, Vol. 1, pp. 1–7. Academic Press, New York.

Ferrier, E., and Davis, M. 1973. A lexical approach to the remediation of final sound omissions. J. Speech Hear. Disord. 38:126–130.

Fey, M. E., and Gandour, J. 1982. Rule discovery in phonological acquisition. J. Child Lang. 9:71–81.

Fisher, H., and Logemann, J. 1971. The Fisher-Logemann Test of Articulation Competence. Houghton Mifflin, Boston.

Fokes, J. 1982. Problems confronting the theorist and practitioner in child phonology. In: M. Crary (ed.), Phonological Intervention—Concepts and Procedures. College-Hill Press, San Diego.

Freeman, F. J. 1982. Prosody in perception, production, and pathologies. In: N. J. Lass (ed.), Speech, Language and Hearing, Vol. 2, pp. 652–671. Saunders, Philadelphia.

Gallagher, T., and Shriner, T. 1975. Contextual variables related to inconsistent /s/ and /z/ production. J. Speech Hear. Res. 18:623–633.

Garnica, O. K. 1973. The development of phonemic speech perception. In: T. E. Moore (ed.), Cognitive Development and the Acquisition of Language, pp. 215–222. Academic Press, New York.

Gesell, A., and **Armatruda, C. S.** 1941. Developmental Diagnosis. Hoeber, New York.

Gleitman, L., and **Wanner, E.** 1982. Language acquisition: The state of the state of the art. In: E. Wanner and L. Gleitman (eds.), Language Acquisition: The State of the Art, pp. 3–48. Cambridge University Press, Cambridge.

Goldman, R., Fristoe, M., and **Woodcock, R.** 1970. The Goldman-Fristoe-Woodcock Test of Auditory Discrimination. American Guidance Service, Circle Pines, MN.

Greenlee, M. 1973. Some observations on initial English consonant clusters in a child two to three years old. Papers Rep. Child Lang. Dev. 6:97–106.

Greenlee, M. 1974. Interacting processes in the child's acquisition of stop-liquid clusters. Papers Rep. Child Lang. Dev. 7:85–100.

Grunwell, P. 1980. Developmental language disorders at the phonological level. In: F. M. Jones (ed.), Language Disability in Children, pp. 129–158. MTP Press, Lancaster, England.

Grunwell, P. 1981. The Nature of Phonological Disability in Children. Academic Press, New York.

Grunwell, P. 1982. Clinical Phonology. Aspen, Rockville, MD.

Haas, W. 1963. Phonological analysis of a case of dyslalia. J. Speech Hear. Disord. 28:239–246.

Halliday, M. A. K. 1975. Learning How to Mean—Explorations in the Development of Language. Edward Arnold, London.

Hargrove, P. 1982. Misarticulated vowels: a case study. Lang. Speech Hear. Serv. Schools 13:86–95.

Hodson, B. 1980. The Assessment of Phonological Processes. The Interstate, Danville, IL.

Hodson, B., and **Paden, E.** 1981. Phonological processes which characterize unintelligible and intelligible speech in early childhood. J. Speech Hear. Disord. 46:369–373.

Hodson, B., and **Paden, E.** 1983. Targeting Intelligible Speech: A Phonological Approach to Remediation. College Hill Press, San Diego.

Hoffman, P., Schuckers, G., and **Daniloff, R.** 1980. Developmental trends in correct /r/ articulation as a function of allophone. J. Speech Hear. Res. 23:746–756.

Hyman, L. 1975. Phonology: Theory and Analysis. Holt, Rinehart & Winston, New York.

Ingram, D. 1974. Fronting in child phonology. J. Child Lang. 1:233–241.

Ingram, D. 1976. Phonological Disability in Children. Edward Arnold, London.

Ingram, D. 1978. The role of the syllable in phonological development. In: A. Bell and J. B. Hooper (eds.), Syllables and Segments, pp. 143–155. North-Holland, Amsterdam.

Ingram, D. 1980. A comparative study of phonological development in normal and linguistically delayed children. Proceedings of the First Wisconsin Symposium on Research in Child Language Disorders, Vol. 1, pp. 23–33.

Ingram, D. 1981. Procedures for the Phonological Analysis of Children's Language. University Park Press, Baltimore.

Ingram, D., Christensen, L., Veach, S., and **Webster, B.** 1980. The acquisition of word-initial fricatives and affricates in English by children between 2 and 6 years. In: G. Yeni-Komshian, J. F. Kavanagh, and C. A. Ferguson (eds.), Child Phonology, Vol. 1, pp. 169–191. Academic Press, New York.

Irwin, J., and **Wong, S.** 1983. Phonological Development in Children 18 to 72 months. Southern Illinois University Press, Carbondale, IL.

Irwin, O. C. 1947. Infant speech: consonantal sounds according to place of articulation. J. Speech Hear. Disord. 12:397–401.

Jakobson, R. 1968. Child Language, Aphasia, and Phonological Universals (A. R. Keiler, trans.). Mouton, The Hague.

Jakobson, R. 1971. Why "mama" and "papa." In: Studies in Child Language and Aphasia, pp. 21–30. Mouton, The Hague.

Jakobson, R., Fant, G., and **Halle, M.** 1963. Preliminaries to Speech Analysis: The Distinctive Features and their Correlates. Technical Report 13, M.I.T. Acoustics Laboratory, 1952. MIT Press, Cambridge, MA.

Jakobson, R., and **Halle, M.** 1956. Fundamentals of Language. Mouton, The Hague.

Jenkins, J. J. 1980. Research in child phonology: comments, criticism, and advice. In: G. Yeni-Komshian, J. F. Kavanagh, and C. A. Ferguson (eds.), Child Phonology, Vol. 2, pp. 217–228. Academic Press, New York.

Johnson, C. J., and **Hardee, P. W.** 1981. Perceptual basis for phonological simplification of the fricative class. Paper presented at the annual meeting of American Speech-Hearing-Language Association, November 19–22, Los Angeles.

Johnson, S., and **Somers, H.** 1978. Spontaneous and imitated responses in articulation testing. Br. J. Disord. Commun. 13:107–116.

Kent, R. 1976. Anatomical and neuromuscular maturation of the speech mechanism: evidence from acoustic studies. J. Speech Hear. Res. 19:421–447.

Kent, R. 1980. Motor skill component of speech development. Paper presented at the annual meeting of the American Speech-Language-Hearing Association, November 21–24, Detroit.

Kent, R. 1981. Articulatory-acoustic perspectives on speech development. In: R. Stark (ed.), Language Behavior in Infancy and Early Childhood, pp. 105–126. Elsevier/North Holland, New York.

Kent, R. 1982. Contextual facilitation of correct sound production. Lang. Speech Hear. Serv. Schools 13:66–76.

Kiparsky, P., and **Menn, L.** 1977. On the acquisition of phonology. In: J. Macnamara (ed.), Language Learning and Thought, pp. 47–78. Academic Press, New York.

Klein, H. B. 1981. Productive strategies for the pronunciation of early polysyllabic lexical items. J. Speech Hear. Res. 24:389–405.

Kornfeld, J. R. 1971. Theoretical issues in child phonology. Papers from the Seventh Regional Meeting of the Chicago Linguistics Society, pp. 454–468.

Kresheck, J. D., and Socolofsky, G. 1972. Imitative and spontaneous articulatory assessment of four-year-old children. J. Speech Hear. Res. 15:729–731.

Kuhl, P. K. 1979. The perception of speech in early infancy. In: N. J. Lass (ed.), Speech and Language: Advances in Basic Research and Practice, Vol. 1, pp. 286–322. Academic Press, New York.

Kuhl, P. K. 1980. Perceptual constancy for speech-sound categories in early infancy. In: G. Yeni-Komshian, J. A. Kavanagh, and C. A. Ferguson (eds.), Child Phonology, Vol. 2, pp. 41–66. Academic Press, New York.

Kuhl, P. K., and Meltzoff, A. 1982. The bimodal perception of speech in infancy. Science 218:1138–1141.

Kuppermann, P., Bligh, S., and Goodban, M. 1980. Activating articulation skills through theraplay. J. Speech Hear. Disord. 45:540–548.

Labov, W., and Labov, T. 1978. The phonetics of cat and mama. Language 54:816–852.

Ladefoged, P. 1971. Preliminaries to Linguistic Phonetics. Chicago University Press, Chicago.

Ladefoged, P. 1975. A Course in Phonetics. Harcourt, Brace, & Jovanovich, New York.

Leonard, L. 1973. The nature of disordered articulation. J. Speech Hear. Disord. 38:156–161.

Leopold, W. F. 1947. Speech Development of a Bilingual Child: A Linguist's Record, Vol. II: Sound-Learning in the First Two Years. Northwestern University, Evanston, IL.

Lieberman, P. 1980. On the development of vowel production in young children. In: G. Yeni-Komshian, J. F. Kavanagh, and C. A. Ferguson (eds.), Child Phonology, Vol. 1, pp. 113–142. Academic Press, New York.

Lieberman, P., Harris, K. S., Wolff, P., and Russell, L. N. 1971. Newborn infant cry and non-human primate vocalizations. J. Speech Hear. Res. 14:718–727.

Locke, J. L. 1980a. The inference of speech perception in the phonologically disordered child. I. A rationale, some criteria, the conventional tests. J. Speech Hear. Disord. 45:431–444.

Locke, J. L. 1980b. The inference of speech perception in the phonologically disordered child. II. Some clinically novel procedures, their use, some findings. J. Speech Hear. Disord. 45:445–468.

Locke, J. L. 1980c. The prediction of child speech errors: Implications for a theory of acquisition. In: G. Yeni-Komshian, J. F. Kavanagh, and C. A. Ferguson (eds.), Child Phonology, Vol. 1, pp. 193–209. Academic Press, New York.

Locke, J. L. 1981. The contributions of adult speech to child speech errors. Mini-seminar presented at the annual meeting of the American Speech-Language-Hearing Association, November 19–22, Los Angeles.

Locke, J. 1983a. Clinical phonology: the explanation and treatment of speech sound disorders. J. Speech Hear. Disord. 48:339–341.

Locke, J. L. 1983b. Phonological Acquisition and Change. Academic Press, New York.

Lorentz, J. 1974. A deviant phonological system of English. Papers Rep. Child Lang. Dev. 8:55–64.

Lorentz, J. 1976. An analysis of some deviant phonological rules of English. In: D. Morehead and A. Morehead (eds.), Normal and Deficient Child Language, pp. 29–59. University Park Press, Baltimore.

Macken, M. A. 1979. Developmental reorganization of phonology: a hierarchy of basic units of acquisition. Lingua 49:11–49.

Macken, M. A. 1980a. Aspects of the acquisition of stop systems: a cross-linguistic perspective. In: G. Yeni-Komshian, J. F. Kavanagh, and C. A. Ferguson (eds.), Child Phonology, Vol. 1, pp. 143–168. Academic Press, New York.

Macken, M. A. 1980b. The child's lexical representation: the "puzzle-puddle-pickle" evidence. J. Linguistics 16:1–17.

Macken, M. A., and Barton, D. 1980. The acquisition of the voicing contrast in English: a study of voice onset time in word-initial stop consonants. J. Child Lang. 7:41–74.

Macken, M. A., and Ferguson, C. A. 1983. Cognitive aspects of phonological development: model, evidence and issues. In: K. E. Nelson (ed.), Children's Language, Vol. 4, pp. 256–282. Erlbaum, Hillsdale, NJ.

Madison, C. 1979. Articulation stimulability reviewed. Lang. Speech Hear. Serv. Schools 10:185–190.

Malsheen, B. J. 1980. Two hypotheses for phonetic clarification in the speech of mothers to children. In: G. Yeni-Komshian, J. F. Kavanagh, and C. A. Ferguson (eds.), Child Phonology, Vol. 2, pp. 173–184. Academic Press, New York.

Martin, F. 1981. Introduction to Audiology. Prentice Hall, Englewood Cliffs, NJ.

Mason, R., and Simon, C. 1977. An orofacial examination checklist. Lang. Speech Hear. Serv. Schools 13:155–163.

Matheny, N., and Panagos, J. 1978. Comparing the effects of articulation and syntax programs on syntax and articulation improvement. Lang., Speech Hear. Serv. Schools 9:57–61.

Maxwell, E. 1982. A study of misarticulation from a linguistic perspective. Doctoral dissertation, MIT, Indiana University Linguistic Club, Bloomington.

Maxwell, E., and Weismer, G. 1982. The contribution of phonological, acoustic, and perceptual techniques to the characterization of a misarticulating child's voice contrast for stops. Appl. Psycholing. 3:29–43.

McDonald, E. 1964. Articulation Testing and Treatment: A Sensory Motor Approach. Stanwix House, Pittsburgh.

McNutt, J. 1977. Oral sensory and motor behaviors of children with /s/ or /r/ misarticulations. J. Speech Hear. Res. 20:694–703.

McReynolds, L., and **Bennett, S.** 1972. Distinctive feature generalization in articulation training. J. Speech Hear. Disord. 37:462–470.

McReynolds, L., and **Elbert, M.** 1981. Generalization of correct articulation in clusters. Appl. Psycholing. 2:119–132.

McReynolds, L., and **Engmann, D.** 1975. Distinctive Feature Analysis of Misarticulations. University Park Press, Baltimore.

McReynolds, L., and **Huston, K.** 1971. A distinctive feature analysis of children's misarticulation. J. Speech Hear. Disord. 39:462–470.

McReynolds, L., **Kohn, J.,** and **Williams, G.** 1975. Articulatory-defective children's discrimination of their production errors. J. Speech Hear. Disord. 40:327–338.

Menn, L. 1976a. Evidence for an interactionist-discovery theory of child phonology. Papers Rep. Child Lang. Dev. 12:169–177.

Menn, L. 1976b. Pattern, control and contrast in beginning speech: a case study in the development of word form and word function. Unpublished doctoral dissertation, University of Illinois.

Menn, L. 1979. Towards a psychology of phonology: child phonology as a first step. In: Proceedings of the Conference on Applications of Linguistic Theory in the Human Sciences. Lansing, MI, pp. 138–179.

Menn, L. 1980. Phonological theory and child phonology. In: G. Yeni-Komshian, J. F. Kavanagh, and C. A. Ferguson (eds.), Child Phonology, Vol. 1, pp. 23–41. Academic Press, New York.

Menn, L. 1982. Theories of phonological development. Ann. N.Y. Acad. Sci. 379:130–137.

Menyuk, P. 1980. The role of context in misarticulation. In: G. Yeni-Komshian, J. F. Kavanagh, and C. A. Ferguson (eds.), Child Phonology, Vol. 1, pp. 211–226. Academic Press, New York.

Menyuk, P., and **Menn, L.** 1979. Early strategies for the perception and production of words and sounds. In: P. Fletcher and M. Garman (eds.), Language Acquisition, pp. 49–70. Cambridge University Press, Cambridge.

Miller, G. A., and **Nicely, P. E.** 1955. An analysis of perceptual confusions among some English consonants. J. Acoust. Soc. Am. 27:338–352.

Miller, J. F. 1981. Assessing Language Production in Children. University Park Press, Baltimore.

Miller, J. F., and **Chapman, R. S.** 1981. The relationship between age and mean length of utterance in morphemes. J. Speech Hear. Res. 24:154–161.

Miller, W., and **Ervin, S.** 1964. The development of grammar in child language. Monogr. Soc. Res. Child Dev. 29(92):9–34.

Morse, P. A. 1972. The discrimination of speech and non-speech stimuli in early infancy. J. Exp. Child Psychol. 14:477–492.

Moskowitz, A. I. 1971. The acquisition of phonology. Unpublished doctoral dissertation, University of California, Berkeley.

Moskowitz, B. A. 1975. The acquisition of fricatives: a study in phonetics and phonology. J. Phonet. 3:141–150.

Moskowitz, B. A. 1980. Idioms in phonology acquisition and phonological change. J. Phonet. 8:69–83.

Mowrer, D. 1977. Methods of Modifying Speech Behaviors, Merrill, Columbus, OH.

Mowrer, O. H. 1952. Speech development in the young child: the autism theory of speech development and some clinical applications. J. Speech Hear. Disord. 17:263–268.

Mowrer, O. H. 1960. Learning Theory and Symbolic Processes. Wiley, New York.

Nakazima, S. A. 1962. A comparative study of the speech developments of Japanese and American English in childhood. Stud. Phonol. 2:27–46.

Nelson, K. 1973. Structure and strategy in learning to talk. Monogr. Soc. Res. Child Dev. 38(149).

Netsell, R. 1981. The acquisition of speech motor control: a perspective with directions for research. In: R. Stark (ed.), Language Behavior in Infancy and Early Childhood, pp. 128–156. Elsevier/North Holland, New York.

Oller, D. K. 1973. Regularities in abnormal child phonology. J. Speech Hear. Disord. 38:36–47.

Oller, D. K. 1980. The emergence of speech sounds in infancy. In: G. Yeni-Komshian, J. A. Kavanagh, and C. A. Ferguson (eds.), Child Phonology, Vol. 1, pp. 93–112. Academic Press, New York.

Oller, D. K., Wieman, L. A., Doyle, W. J., and Ross, C. 1976. Infant babbling and speech. J. Child Lang. 3:1–11.

Olmsted, D. 1966. A theory of the child's learning of phonology. Language 42:531–535.

Olmsted, D. 1971. Out of the Mouth of Babes. Mouton, The Hague.

Olney, R. L., and Scholnick, E. K. 1976. Adult judgments of age and linguistic differences in infant vocalization. J. Child Lang. 3:145–155.

Olswang, L., and Bain, B. 1982. Criteria for sound mastery: when can treatment be terminated? Paper presented at the American Speech-Language-Hearing Association Convention, November 18–21, Toronto.

Pačesova, J. 1968. The Development of Vocabulary in the Child. J. E. Purkyne, Brno Universita.

Panagos, J. 1978. Abstract phonology, grammatical reduction and delayed speech development. Acta Symbol. 7:1–12.

Panagos, J., Quine, M., and Klich, R. 1979. Syntactic and phonological influences on children's articulation. J. Speech Hear. Res. 22:841–848.

Parker, F. 1976. Distinctive features in speech pathology: phonology or phonemics? J. Speech Hear. Disord. 41:23–39.

Paynter, E. T., and Bumpas, T. C. 1977. Imitative and spontaneous articulatory assessment of three-year-old children. J. Speech Hear. Disord. 42:119–125.

Peters, A. M. 1983. The Units of Language Acquisition. Cambridge Monographs and Texts in Applied Psycholinguistics. Cambridge Univeresity Press, Cambridge.

Poole, I. 1934. Genetic development of articulation of consonant sounds in speech. Elementary English Rev. 11:159–161.

Powers, M. H. 1957. Clinical and educational procedures in functional disorders of articulation. In: L. Travis (ed.), Handbook of Speech Pathology and Audiology, pp. 707–768. Appleton-Century-Crofts, New York.

Powers, M. 1971. Clinical and educational procedures in functional disorders of articulation. In: L. Travis (ed.), Handbook of Speech Pathology and Audiology, pp. 877–910. Appleton-Century-Crofts, New York.

Prather, E. M., Hedrick, D. L., and **Kern, C. A.** 1975. Articulation development in children aged two to four years. J. Speech Hear. Disord. 40:179–191.

Priestly, T. M. S. 1977. One idiosyncratic strategy in the acquisition of phonology. J. Child Lang. 4:45–66.

Renfrew, C. 1966. Persistence of the open syllable in defective articulation. J. Speech Hear. Disord. 31:370–373.

Ruder, K., and **Bunce, B.** 1981. Articulation therapy using distinctive feature analysis to structure the training program: two case studies. J. Speech Hear. Disord. 46:59–65.

Ruscello, D., and **Shelton, R.** 1979. Planning and self-assessment in articulatory training. J. Speech Hear. Disord. 44:504–512.

Sander, E. 1972. When are speech sounds learned? J. Speech Hear. Disord. 37:55–63.

Schwartz, R. G., and **Leonard, L. B.** 1982. Do children pick and choose? An examination of phonological selection and avoidance in early lexical acquisition. J. Child Lang. 9:319–336.

Schwartz, R., Leonard, L., Folger, M., and **Wilcox, M.** 1980. Early phonological behavior in normal-speaking and language-disordered children: evidence for a synergistic view of linguistic disorders. J. Speech Hear. Disord. 45:357–377.

Scollon, R. 1976. Conversations with a One Year Old. The University of Hawaii Press, Honolulu.

Shelton, R., and **McReynolds, L.** 1979. Functional articulation disorders: preliminaries to treatment. In: N. Lass (ed.), Speech and Language Advances in Basic Research and Practice, Vol. 2, pp. 1–111. Academic Press, New York.

Shibamoto, J. S., and **Olmsted, D.** 1978. Lexical and syllabic patterns in phonological acquisition. J. Child Lang. 5:417–457.

Shriberg, L. 1982a. Diagnostic assessment of developmental phonological disorders. In: M. Crary (ed.), Phonological Intervention—Concepts and Procedures, pp. 35–60. College Hill Press, San Diego.

Shriberg, L. 1982b. Programming for the language component in developmental phonological disorders. Semin. Speech, Lang. Hear. 3:115–126.

Shriberg, L., and **Kent, R.** 1982. Clinical Phonetics. Wiley, New York.

Shriberg, L., and **Kwiatkowski, J.** 1980. Natural Process Analysis: A Procedure for Phonological Analysis of Continuous Speech Samples. Wiley, New York.

Shriberg, L., and **Kwiatkowski, J.** 1982a. Phonological disorders. II. A conceptual framework for management. J. Speech Hear. Disord. 47:242–256.

Shriberg, L., and **Kwiatkowski, J.** 1982b. Phonological disorders. III. A procedure for assessing severity of involvement. J. Speech Hear. Disord. 47:256–270.

Shvachkin, N. K. 1973. The development of phonemic speech perception in early childhood. In: C. A. Ferguson, and D. I. Slobin (eds.), Studies of Child Language Development, pp. 91–127. Holt, Rinehart, and Winston, New York.

Siegel, G., Winitz, H., and **Conkey, H.** 1963. The influence of testing instruments on articulatory responses of children. J. Speech Hear. Disord. 28:67–76.

Singh, S., and **Polen, S.** 1972. Use of distinctive feature model in speech pathology. Acta Symbol. 3:17–25.

Sloat, C., Taylor, S. H. and **Hoard, J.** 1978. Introduction to Phonology. Prentice-Hall, Englewood Cliffs, NJ.

Slobin, D. I. 1982. Universals and particulars in the acquisition of language. In: E. Wanner and L. R. Gleitman (eds.), Language Acquisition: The State of the Art, pp. 128–170. Cambridge University Press, Cambridge.

Smith, B. L. 1978. Temporal aspects of speech productions: a developmental perspective. J. Phonet. 6:37–68.

Smith, B. L. 1979. A phonetic analysis of consonantal devoicing in children's speech. J. Child Lang. 6:19–28.

Smith, B. L. 1981. Explaining the development of speech production skills in young children. J. Nat. Student Speech Lang. Hear. Assoc. 9:9–19.

Smith, B. L., and **Oller, D. K.** 1981. A comparative study of pre-meaningful vocalizations produced by normally developing and Down's syndrome infants. J. Speech Hear. Disord. 46:46–51.

Smith, N. V. 1973. The Acquisition of Phonology: A Case Study. Cambridge University Press, Cambridge.

Snow, C. E., and **Ferguson, C. A.** 1977. Talking to Children: Language Input and Acquisition. Cambridge University Press, Cambridge.

Snow, K. 1963. A detailed analysis of articulation responses of "normal" first grade children. J. Speech Hear. Res. 6:277–290.

Spring, D. R., and **Dale, P. S.** 1975. Discrimination of stress in early infancy. J. Speech Hear. Res. 20:224–231.

St. Louis, K., and **Ruscello, D.** 1981. The Oral Speech Mechanism Screening Examination. University Park Press, Baltimore.

Stampe, D. 1969. The acquisition of phonetic representation. Papers from the Fifth Regional Meeting of the Chicago Linguistic Society, 433–444. Chicago Linguistic Society, Chicago.

Stampe, D. 1973. A dissertation on natural phonology. Unpublished doctoral dissertation, University of Chicago.

Stark, R. E. 1978. Features of infant sounds: the emergence of cooing. J. Child Lang. 5:379–390.

Stoel-Gammon, C. 1981. Final report for research grant NIH-NICHD

5-R01-HD-1295. Aspects of Normal and Abnormal Phonological Development.

Stoel-Gammon, C. 1983a. Constraints on consonant-vowel sequences in early words. J. Child Lang. 10:455–457.

Stoel-Gammon, C. 1983b. Variations of style in mothers' speech to young children. Paper presented at the annual convention of the American Speech-Language-Hearing Association, November 18–21, Cincinnati.

Stoel-Gammon, C. 1984. Phonetic inventories, 15–24 months: a longitudinal study. Paper presented at the Third International Congress for the Study of Child Language, July 8–13, Austin, TX.

Stoel-Gammon, C., and Cooper, J. 1981. Individual differences in early phonological and lexical development. Paper presented at the Second International Congress for the Study of Child Language, August 9–14, Vancouver, BC.

Stoel-Gammon, C., and Cooper, J. 1984. Patterns of early lexical and phonological development. J. Child Lang. 11:247–271.

Stoel-Gammon, C., Smith, B. L., and Minifie, F. D. 1978. Analyzing phonological development: computer applications. Scientific exhibit presented at the annual convention of the American Speech-Language-Hearing Association, November 18–21, San Francisco.

Stokes, T., and Baer, D. 1977. An implicit technology of generalization. J. Appl. Behav. Anal. 10:349–367.

Straight, H. S. 1980. Auditory versus articulatory phonological processes and their development in children. In: G. Yeni-Komshian, J. A. Kavanagh, and C. A. Ferguson (eds.), Child Phonology, Vol. 1, pp. 43–71. Academic Press, New York.

Strange, W., and Broen, P. A. 1980. Perception and production of approximant consonants by 3-year-olds: a first study. In: G. Yeni-Komshian, J. Kavanagh, and C. Ferguson (eds.), Child Phonology, Vol. 2, pp. 117–154. Academic Press, New York.

Templin, M. C. 1947. Spontaneous versus imitated verbalization in testing articulation in preschool children. J. Speech Hear. Disord. 18:293–300.

Templin, M. C. 1957. Certain Language Skills in Children: Their Development and Interrelationships. Institute of Child Welfare Monographs, Vol. 26. University of Minnesota Press, Minneapolis.

Templin, M. C., and Darley, F. L. 1960. The Templin-Darley tests of articulation. Bureau of Educational Research and Service Extension Division, Iowa City.

Tiffany, W., and Carrell, J. 1977. Phonetics: Theory and Application. McGraw-Hill, New York.

Tingley, B. M., and Allen, G. D. 1975. Development of speech timing control in children. Child Dev. 46:186–194.

Uzgiris, I., and Hunt, J. 1975. Assessment in Infancy: Ordinal Scales of Psychological Development. University of Illinois Press, Urbana.

Van Riper, C. 1972. Speech Correction: Principles and Methods, 5th Ed. Prentice-Hall, Englewood Cliffs, NJ.

Velten, H. V. 1943. The growth of phonemic and lexical patterns in infant language. Language 19:281–292.

Vihman, M. 1978. Consonant harmony: Its scope and function in child language. In: J. Greenberg, C. A. Ferguson, and E. A. Moravcsik (eds.), Universals of Human Language, Vol. 2, pp. 281–334. Stanford University Press, Stanford, CA.

Vihman, M. 1981. Phonology and the development of the lexicon. J. Child Lang. 8:239–265.

Vihman, M., Macken, M. A., Miller, R., and **Simmons, H.** 1981. From babbling to speech: a reassessment of the continuity issue. Paper presented at the annual meeting of the Linguistic Society of America, December, New York.

Walsh, H. 1974. On certain practical inadequacies of distinctive feature systems. J. Speech Hear. Disord. 39:32–43.

Wang, M. D., and **Bilger, R. C.** 1973. Consonant confusions in noise: a study of perceptual features. J. Acoust. Soc. Am. 54:1248–1266.

Waterson, N. 1970. Some speech forms of an English child: a phonological study. Transactions of the Philological Society, 1–24.

Waterson, N. 1971. Child phonology: a prosodic view. J. Linguistics 7:179–211.

Weiner, F. 1979. Phonological Process Analysis. University Park Press, Baltimore.

Weiner, F. 1981a. Systematic sound preference as a characteristic of phonological disability. J. Speech Hear. Disord. 46:281–286.

Weiner, F. 1981b. Treatment of phonological disability using the method of meaningful minimal contrast: two case studies. J. Speech Hear. Disord. 46:97–103.

Weiner, F., and **Bankson, N.** 1978. Teaching features. Lang. Speech Hear. Serv. Schools 9:29–34.

Weir, R. H. 1962. Language in the Crib. Mouton, The Hague.

Wellman, B. L., Case, I. M., Mengert, I. G., and **Bradbury, D. E.** 1931. Speech sounds of young children. Univ. Iowa Stud. Child Welfare 5(2).

Wepman, J. 1973. Wepman Auditory Discrimination Test. Language Research Associates, Chicago.

Westby, C. 1980. Assessment of cognitive and language abilities through play. Lang. Speech Hear. Serv. Schools 11:154–168.

Williams, G., and **McReynolds, L.** 1975. The relationship between discrimination and articulation training in children with misarticulations. J. Speech Hear. Res. 18:401–412.

Winitz, H. 1969. Articulatory Acquisition and Behavior. Prentice-Hall, Englewood Cliffs, NJ.

Winitz, H. 1975. From Syllable to Conversation. University Park Press, Baltimore.

Winitz, H., and **Irwin, O. C.** 1958. Syllabic and phonetic structure of infants' early words. J. Speech Hear. Res. 1:250–256.

Yeni-Komshian, G., Kavanagh, J. F., and Ferguson, C. A. (eds.). 1980. Child Phonology. Vols. 1 and 2. Academic Press, New York.

Zlatin, M. A. 1974. Variations on a theme: [agɣʊə] Paper presented the American Speech and Hearing Association Convention, November, Las Vegas.

Index

A

Acoustic analysis of speech sounds, 4, 8, 97, 102, 104, 119

Acquisition of phonology, 3, 15–74
see also Development, phonological

Adult speech, compared to child's productions, 87–88
see also Relational analysis

Advanced forms in phonological development, 53, 54, 86, 198

Affricates, 9
  acquisition of, 30, 46, 48, 63, 64
    position within word affecting, 32
  articulatory difficulty of, 48
  in disordered phonology, 135, 147, 158
  independent analysis of, 90, 99
  prelinguistic, 19
  relational analysis of, 93, 147, 158
  substitution errors concerning, 40

Age, and phonological development, 196
  in customary production of consonantal phonemes, 31
  in mastery of consonantal phonemes, 30, 31, 32, 33
  in phonological processes, 42–45
  in relation to disordered phonology, 121

Allophones, 10
  in complementary distribution, 10
  in free variation, 10

Alveolars, 9, 11, 12
  acquisition of, 46
  assimilation of, in disordered phonology, 158
  in first words, 23
  substitution errors concerning, 40, 46

Analysis of speech sounds, 8–11, 85–89
  see also Assessment procedures

Articulatory features
  acquisition of, 3, 4, 46
  motor ability for, 3, 6

225